W9-BMW-182

What is a Christian to think when a loved one who has been faithful to God's commands and steeped in his Word behaves in ways that are strange to family and even to self? Do we fear ourselves that we may lose our memory, our mind, such that all spiritual that we value dissolves into apparent oblivion? Ben Mast has provided us with much-needed perspective and encouragement about the ongoing interaction among God, family, and those who begin to forget.

DAN G. BLAZER, MD, MPH, PhD, JP Gibbons Professor of Psychiatry and
Behavioral Sciences, Duke University Medical Center, Durham, NC

My mother, one the godliest people to ever walk on this earth, died from Alzheimer's. The debilitating effects of this disease were almost more than we could bear. A book like this would have been worth its weight in gold! I cannot commend highly enough what a gift it will be to families everywhere.

DANIEL L. AKIN, President, Southeastern Baptist
Theological Seminary, Wake Forest, NC

We forget … God always remembers. Thank you, Ben, for this profound reminder.

JOLENE BRACKEY, national speaker on Alzheimer's Disease,
author of *Creating Moments of Joy*

With pastoral tenderness and gospel confidence, Mast shepherds the readers to see how Alzheimer's Disease cannot and will not have the final say as our faithful God will not forget us. Second Forgetting is a gift to the church as it serves as an essential resource to equip the body of Christ to care for one another with the gospel during times of deep suffering.

ROBERT K. CHEONG, Pastor of Care, Sojourn
Community Church, Louisville, KY

One of the greatest fears of growing old is the ever-increasing possibility of developing Alzheimer's or another dementia, raising the lament, "Who am I if I can't remember who I am?" Using Scripture and inspiring testimonies of dementia-afflicted people he has known and helped, Dr. Mast shows the reader how to respond to the experience of dementia as God's beloved children.

JANE M. THIBAULT, PhD, Clinical Professor Emerita, Clinical Gerontologist,
University of Louisville, School of Medicine

Second Forgetting isn't simply scientific theories regarding the brain, Alzheimer's, and memory loss, but the deep, prayerful, and careful counsel of a pastor. Dr. Mast is not only a seasoned scholar but a soul physician. My hope is that his prescription would lead to a healthier, holier and more hopeful church. Buy this book.

> DANIEL MONTGOMERY, Pastor of Sojourn Community Church,
> Louisville, KY; author of *Faithmapping and PROOF: Finding
> Freedom through the Intoxicating Joy of Irresistible Grace*

When memory is compromised we lose touch with connections to people … and also with God. Benjamin Mast takes us into the inside of memory loss and helps us understand from within what it is like to experience such a tragic, disabling disease. Caregivers who read this book will respond more empathically and effectively to people who struggle to remember.

> RONALD J. NYDAM, PhD, DMin, Professor of Pastoral Care,
> Calvin Theological Seminary; Author of *Adoptees
> Come of Age: Living Within Two Families*

Dr. Mast leads the reader through *Second Forgetting* to Second Remembering as he reminds us that all people have infinite value and that God remembers each person no matter the circumstances. This book contains a powerful message of hope, written especially for those of the Christian faith, but it also contains eternal truths helpful for individuals of all faiths. This message is a must for those of us dedicated to a better way of communicating and relating to the person with dementia.

> VIRGINIA BELL, MSW, co-author of
> *The Best Friends Approach* books

An expert in the field of Alzheimer's, Mast has woven together the latest research with a gospel-centered orientation and the compassion of a caregiver to produce a biblically informed and practical guide for those in the early stages of the disease and those who love or minister to those afflicted. A welcome and needed resource!

> ERIC JOHNSON, Professor of Pastoral Care, The Southern Baptist Theological
> Seminary, and Director of the Society for Christian Psychology

SECOND FORGETTING

REMEMBERING THE POWER OF THE GOSPEL
DURING ALZHEIMER'S DISEASE

DR. BENJAMIN MAST

FOREWORD BY SCOTTY SMITH

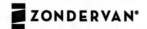

ZONDERVAN

Second Forgetting
Copyright © 2014 by Benjamin T. Mast

This title is also available as a Zondervan ebook.
Visit www.zondervan.com/ebooks.

Requests for information should be addressed to:

Zondervan, 3900 *Sparks Drive SE, Grand Rapids, Michigan 49546*

Library of Congress Cataloging-in-Publication Data

Mast, Benjamin T.
   Second forgetting : remembering the power of the gospel during Alzheimer's
   disease / Dr. Benjamin Mast.
      pages cm
   ISBN 978-0-310-51387-2 (softcover)
      1. Alzheimer's disease—Patients—Religious life. 2. Caregivers—Religious life.
   3. Alzheimer's disease—Religious aspects—Christianity. 4. Caring—Religious
   aspects—Christianity. I. Title.
   BV4910.6.A55M37 2014
   259'.4196831—dc23   2014001199

Cover design: IMAGO
Cover photography: Shutterstock
Interior design and composition: Greg Johnson/Textbook Perfect

Printed in the United States of America

14 15 16 17 18 19 20 /DCI/ 21 20 19 18 17 16 15 14 13 12 11 10 9 8 7 6 5 4 3 2 1

This book is dedicated to those who feel forgotten...
and was written to remind you that you are not.

CONTENTS

FOREWORD

"DAD, IT'S ME, SCOTTY ... YOUR YOUNGEST SON."

I never thought I'd have to say those words — words pregnant with pain and sadness. I was still learning to accept the fact that my dad no longer recognized me. He had forgotten my face. He had forgotten my name. And this forgetting was far more difficult than I had expected. I just couldn't wrap my head and heart around it. Nothing had prepared me for this new chapter in life, learning to love and care for a father who could no longer remember his own son.

I shouldn't have been surprised, though. After all, there is dementia and Alzheimer's on both sides of my family. So there is a very real possibility that I too will one day forget the people I love most in this world. Walking through Alzheimer's with my father made me think about that and wonder: is there anything I can do to, in faith and not fear, to prepare for this possibility?

I wish Ben's book had been published a decade earlier, but even so, I am *so* thankful to have it now. Benjamin Mast is a man who is trained as a scientist and clinician, and who loves the gospel. What a gift, what a treasure, what a compendium of hope and wisdom I've found *Second Forgetting* to be! As a pastor, I now have a medically sensitive, gospel-saturated book to share with those under my care, one that I can recommend to a wide audience of family and friends, to anyone who might be impacted by the issue of memory loss. In addition, I now have an incredible tool to prepare me for the unknown challenges I may one day face should I begin to suffer from significant memory impairment.

During the later stages of my dad's illness, there was one verse of Scripture that I pondered more than any other, Isaiah 49:15: "Can a mother forget the baby at her breast and have no compassion on the child she has borne? Though she may forget, I will not forget you!" As I read this book, Ben brought this text alive for me in several profound ways. On one hand, he gave me fresh insight into the incredibly good news that God is compassionate and does not forget those he loves. No matter *what* goes on in the complex world of our memories, God will *never* forget us — he will never suffer confusion or memory loss.

Even with regard to our sin, God doesn't suffer amnesia as some commonly suggest. He *grace*-fully chooses *not* to remember our sins against us, instead remembering (accounting and applying) Christ's righteousness to us. What peace and freedom this brings! It is yet another way of celebrating the good news that God's grip on us, in the gospel, is much more important than our grasp of the gospel. God's love is the only love that will *never* let go of us. We're not saved by our own memory; we are saved by the God who remembers us, by the memory of a great God of grace and mercy.

Secondly, Ben helped me to recognize the importance of exercising my brainpower right now, while I still can. As he points out in this book, short-term memory is the first thing "to go" when a person suffers from dementia, but our deepest and most treasured memories will tend to stay with us the longest. I saw firsthand how true this was in caring for my dad.

Dad loved and celebrated his life as a navigator in the merchant marines. Having grown up in a violent and extremely poor family in Danville, Virginia, dad escaped the dark vortex of life when he joined the Navy, and then, years later, graduated from the Merchant Marine Academy. Through the course of his career, he navigated ships to sixty different countries, reading the stars and charting a course with only a sextant. Long after my dad failed to recall my face and name, he could still recall amazing stories of his time on the high seas and the exotic ports he had visited. It is the things that we treasure and rehearse most often that tend to stay with us the longest.

This is why, in the spirit of the great German reformer Martin Luther, Ben reminds us that we need to hear the gospel *every* day. Even if we aren't struggling with dementia or Alzheimer's, we still have a natural tendency to forget the gospel. Ben encourages us to feed and feast on the good news of God's grace — to meditate and ruminate upon this truth. The deeper our "memory roots" are established in the gospel, the greater its long-term impact will be.

Second Forgetting is more than just an outstanding introduction to the brain, Alzheimer's, and the physical symptoms of memory loss. It's more than a helpful guide and encouragement for those engaged in compassionate caregiving. It's also a gracious appeal to each of us to become more thoroughly aware of the riches of the gospel, committed to growing in the grace and knowledge of our Lord and Savior, Jesus Christ.

I cannot overstate how wise, kind, and hope filled this book is. I know that I will buy and give out copies in droves. Thank you, Ben, for stewarding God's gospel — and good science — so very well.

Scotty Smith,
West End Community Church

PREFACE

THIS IS A BOOK ABOUT HOPE.

There *is* hope in Alzheimer's disease, but it isn't where most people look for it. I wrote this book for people with Alzheimer's disease and other dementias, and for their families, so that they might reconnect with the power and hope of the gospel. I also wrote it for the church, so that Christians might have a clearer vision for how to care for those in these circumstances of life. Although much of this book is focused on Alzheimer's disease, the truths of Scripture are relevant to other forms of cognitive and behavioral change in later life.

Dementia is a broad term that reflects mental decline, particularly later in life. Alzheimer's and dementia are not the same thing. Dementia is the broader umbrella category, with Alzheimer's being one type of dementia (just as leukemia is one type of cancer). Alzheimer's disease is by far the most common form of dementia, but there are many other forms that share symptoms with Alzheimer's; these include vascular dementia, dementia with Lewy bodies, Parkinson's dementia, frontotemporal dementia, and other rare conditions such as progressive supranuclear palsy. All of these conditions affect our ability to think and remember. Although Alzheimer's and dementia are not exactly the same thing, I use those terms interchangeably throughout this book because most of the material is relevant to both.

This book seeks to communicate hope and encouragement to anyone who has trouble remembering, regardless of the cause.

Finally, this book is written for anyone who has trouble remembering, even if that person's brain is relatively healthy. By considering how we can help other people remember, we also learn how we can better remember the Lord, what he has done, and his promises.

In this book you'll read the stories of those I've met who continue to cling to the power and hope of the gospel despite tremendous challenges and suffering. Their stories demonstrate the reality of holding on to Christ when everything else seems to be slipping away.

Chapter 1

WHAT IS THE SECOND FORGETTING?

LEWIS HAS BEEN RETIRED FOR JUST A YEAR AND A HALF. He worked in home construction and then as a handyman for decades. Because he loves golf and travel, he worked past age sixty-five so he could save up enough money to be able to visit golf courses along the coast. He and his wife, Ann, had just visited one course in North Carolina and had a wonderful time. The weather was perfect, Lewis had more birdies than bogies, and they ended each day with a glass of wine on the beach. It was everything they had hoped retirement would be—until Ann noticed something that made her uneasy.

Lewis had always had a habit of recounting his successes on the course—a powerful drive or a long putt that almost dropped. In all honesty, Ann wasn't usually interested. They all seemed similar, so she often gave the appearance of listening while her attention was elsewhere, whether a magazine or the sunset. But she will never forget this night because there was something in the way he told the story that caught her attention.

On the last hole Lewis had teed off, hoping to hit the green. As he told the story, he knew he'd hit the ball well and saw it soar over a small hill toward the green. As he walked over that hill he was surprised to find the ball sitting mere inches from the flag. His heart had thumped as he realized he had almost hit his first hole in one. Back at the hotel, his excitement was apparent, and Ann knew she'd be hearing about this for quite some time. Sure enough, he talked about it as they got dressed for dinner and brought it up again at dinner and even mentioned it to their waiter. He was proud, and she understood this was part of the enjoyment of the game for him, so his talking about it over and over made sense.

But as they sat on the beach at sunset, he told the story again. She couldn't say exactly how, but there was something slightly different in the way he told it, almost as if he didn't realize he had already told her the whole story several times. Her heart rate quickened. She knew Lewis's mom had suffered with Alzheimer's, for she and Lewis had spent countless hours taking care of her in her later years when she had become unable to care for herself. Lewis's mom had developed the habit of repeating herself early on, and this only stopped when she became unable to speak much at all. As Ann recalled those days, she began to feel overwhelmed. Was Lewis heading down the same road? Ann couldn't help but focus on this repetition as Lewis finished his story again, but she eventually talked herself out of jumping to conclusions. She remained quiet and just listened.

Eventually Ann thought about other things, and they continued their journey with great enjoyment—until a month later when she became concerned again. Lewis had arranged to meet with some friends in a nearby city. He and a friend golfed in the afternoon and met up with their wives for dinner. Ann noticed that he was unusually quiet during dinner and seemed to have trouble deciding what to order. Then he leaned over to Ann and said, "I'm going to the men's room. Can you order me something good?" He gave her a quick smile and a kiss on the cheek before departing. Lewis had always been particular about his food, so this struck her as odd, but it didn't raise her concern until Lewis's friend spoke.

"Ann, I feel a bit awkward asking this, but we've been friends for a long time, and ... well ... how's Lewis doing?"

Ann's heart jumped, and once again she found herself becoming overwhelmed with a growing fear of what might be coming. "What do you mean?"

"Well, it's probably nothing, but he seems different. I know we haven't seen you in a while, but Lewis just seems more quiet than usual, and when we golfed today, a couple of times I could have sworn he was getting stuck on certain words. On one hole he asked me to bring him 'that club'; I knew he needed his putter because he was on the green, but it struck me as strange. I know he's not as young as he used to be, and I don't want to pick on him, but his mother had dementia or something, and I couldn't help but notice that he seemed a little foggy. When we got back to the clubhouse, he was a little confused about where to go. Again, I'm not sure, it was a new course for him, but it's just not like him ... you know?"

Unfortunately, she did. She had been debating with herself about whether to push Lewis to talk to his doctor, but at this moment, the debate ended. A few days later she asked him — then pleaded with him — to make an appointment.

Ann's talk with Lewis hadn't gone well. She'd been uncertain about what to say and when to say it, and when she finally brought up the subject, he downplayed his forgetfulness and dismissed her concerns. But she was worried, so she continued to press him. Eventually he became angry and shouted at her, speaking words that she hadn't heard him speak in decades.

Three months later, they walked into the doctor's exam room together. Lewis and the doctor discussed the weather, their golf games, and other matters until Ann couldn't stand it any longer. Was Lewis going to say anything about his memory? Was the doctor going to get down to business? She finally broke in with a list of things that she had observed that concerned her — the repetition of stories, the forgetfulness of events and conversations, his difficulty thinking of the words, and his trouble with directions.

Soon the doctor began testing. He asked Lewis some questions, which to Ann seemed much too easy. The doctor asked about the date, the day of the week, and the year. Lewis got these correct, though Ann was surprised to see him struggle a little. When the doctor pointed to his wristwatch and asked Lewis what it was called, Lewis hesitated and the room grew unusually quiet. Five seconds seemed like five minutes. Finally, Lewis said, "This is silly kid's stuff." He couldn't remember what a watch was called. A short time later the doctor asked him to recall three words he had been instructed to remember earlier in the exam. He couldn't even remember one of them. Tears welled up in Ann's eyes, but she pushed them back so her husband wouldn't see.

Lewis was clearly having difficulty remembering things, and as it turned out, it was caused by Alzheimer's, a frightening disease characterized by progressively worsening memory. His forgetting had grown increasingly obvious—once Alzheimer's grabs hold, the forgetting is unmistakable and sometimes terrifying.

The initial forgetting of Alzheimer's is a subtle, gradual onset, getting steadily worse over time. It signals that something might be wrong and causes family members like Ann to be concerned. Doctors and other healthcare professionals focus much of their effort on evaluating this form of forgetting to determine whether a person has Alzheimer's disease or another condition of aging. The Alzheimer's Association estimates that over $200 billion are spent annually on Alzheimer's care.

As Lewis and Ann listened to the doctor deliver the Alzheimer's diagnosis, a second forgetting began to creep in. This second forgetting took hold as they considered the magnitude of what they were facing.

The Second Forgetting

We are all imperfect and broken. We forget the Lord, even in the best of health. This is what I call "the second forgetting." The first forgetting is experienced by the person with Alzheimer's, but the second forgetting reflects a spiritual forgetting experienced not only by the person with Alzheimer's, but more broadly by their family, friends, and even the church who seeks to care for them.

To understand such second forgetting we need to consider a story about an entire community that was prone to forget. The story is much older than Lewis and Ann, but it shares some similarity with theirs. The story is about the people of Israel in the Old Testament who, like Lewis and Ann, were prone to forget the Lord.

> The second forgetting reflects a spiritual forgetting experienced not only by the person with Alzheimer's, but more broadly by their family, friends, and even the church who seeks to care for them.

God had made a promise to a man named Abraham, a promise to make him a great nation, to give the people of Israel a Promised Land of rest, and to be with them always (Genesis 12, 17). But after several generations, they found themselves enslaved and subjected to oppressive forced labor in a foreign land (Exodus 1). They groaned under their suffering and saw no hope of rescue or deliverance. The promises God made to Abraham were far from their minds, and to them it must have seemed they had no hope.

But God heard his people groaning and delivered this message:

> I am the LORD. I appeared to Abraham, to Isaac and to Jacob as God Almighty, but by my name the LORD I did not make myself fully known to them. I also established my covenant with them to give them the land of Canaan, where they resided as foreigners. Moreover, I have heard the groaning of the Israelites, whom the Egyptians are enslaving, and I have remembered my covenant.
>
> Therefore, say to the Israelites: "I am the LORD, and I will bring you out from under the yoke of the Egyptians. I will free you from being slaves to them, and I will redeem you with an outstretched arm and with mighty acts of judgment. I will take you as my own people, and I will be your God. Then you will know that I am the LORD your God, who brought you out from under the yoke of the Egyptians. And I will bring you to the land I swore with uplifted hand to give to Abraham, to Isaac and to Jacob. I will give it to you as a possession. I am the LORD." (Exodus 6:2–8)

In the midst of their suffering, God had heard the groaning of his people and remembered and reaffirmed his promises—to deliver them, be with them, and bring them into the Promised Land. Suffering is a part of this world. It was present during the ancient days of Israel, and it will be present until the Lord brings full restoration. While his people wait, they cry out to God. When God's children groan, God *remembers* his promise and responds.

Even so, because their suffering was so great, the people of Israel did not listen to the great promises of God. Although they didn't listen and remember, God followed through on his promises. He heard their groans and took clear steps to rescue them, and these steps were not subtle (see the story of the plagues in Exodus 7–11). Finally, Pharaoh relented and the Israelites were set free, only to be chased again when Pharaoh changed his mind. But God rescued the Israelites by parting the Red Sea.

After their deliverance, they celebrated with song:

> *The LORD is my strength and my defense;*
> *he has become my salvation.*
> *He is my God, and I will praise him,*
> *my father's God, and I will exalt him....*
> *Who among the gods*
> *is like you, LORD?*
> *Who is like you—*
> *majestic in holiness,*
> *awesome in glory,*
> *working wonders?...*
> *In your unfailing love you will lead*
> *the people you have redeemed.*
> *In your strength you will guide them*
> *to your holy dwelling.*
> *(Exodus 15:2, 11, 13)*

It was a truly unforgettable moment. God remembered his promise, reminded his people of that promise, and miraculously delivered them. It seems that all this would forever be etched in the minds of the Israelites with the faithfulness of God. How could they ever doubt God or complain about his provision again? Certainly, they would never forget!

Yet it only took three days for Israel to forget what God had done.

They grumbled against God and doubted his provision because they couldn't find water. Despite their grumbling, God was gracious and took care of their needs — providing water to drink, and eventually manna and quail to eat.

So a cycle emerges. It starts with God promising to be among his people, to care for them, and to deliver them to the home he has promised. Next, the Israelites face difficulties and suffering, and they forget God and doubt these promises. They groan under the weight of their suffering. God hears them and remembers his promises, and finally, God delivers them (although not always as soon as they would like), continuing to be faithful to what he has promised. This is sometimes followed by a period of rejoicing, but eventually new difficulties emerge and a new cycle begins. With each new difficulty they forget his faithfulness and begin to groan and grumble.

The fact that we rejoice in God's goodness one minute and grumble against him in the next reflects the brokenness of our memory and our ongoing struggle with sin. God knows our need for reminders. He asked Moses to bottle up some manna as a reminder for future generations (Exodus 16:32). Later, God tells Moses to record their victory in battle "as something to be remembered" and pass it on to Joshua, the leader of the next generation. God knows the tendency of his people to forget him and his faithfulness. He encourages them to retain reminders so that this remembrance can be passed down to encourage the faith of his people and to bring them the assurance of his presence when they are suffering.

This cycle was on full display when they were eventually led to the brink of the Promised Land. God had brought them through so much and had now delivered them to the land he had promised them. He had never failed to deliver on his promises, and this seemed to be the culmination. God showed them the land and told them to take it. But instead of remembering his promises and faithfulness in the past, they only saw a new threat. Instead of trusting God's promises and responding in faith, they became fearful and decided to check it out for themselves. They sent out ten spies. Most of them returned with reports of how powerful the people in the land appeared and how easily they could defeat the Israelites. Only two spies dissented, trusting in God and remembering his faithfulness in the past and his promises for the future.

When we are faced with threats, where do our minds go? Do we focus on the magnitude of the threat or on the remembrance of God's past faithfulness and his promises for the future? When we focus on the threat, we begin to forget. That's what Israel did, and that's what God's people have been doing for thousands of years since. The people resumed their grumbling, saying that God had only led them there to die. Despite God's previous rescue and grace-filled care, they seemed to forget and refused to believe in his goodness and faithfulness. Functionally, they forgot the Lord, and wandering in the wilderness soon followed.

Still, this was not the end of God's promise. He always remembers and never fails to deliver. After forty years God led them back to the Promised Land, this time with a warning and another explicit call to remember. In Deuteronomy the Israelites are commanded to remember their wandering in the desert, the way God provided for them with manna, and his promise to deliver them into the Promised Land. In fact, much of the book of Deuteronomy is Moses' remembrance and retelling of the story of the nation of Israel and their trials leading up to the entry into Canaan. When the Israelites were faced with great fear, they heard these words:

> You may say to yourselves, "These nations are stronger than we are. How can we drive them out?" But do not be afraid of them; remember well what the LORD your God did to Pharaoh and to all Egypt. You saw with your own eyes the great trials, the signs and wonders, the mighty hand and outstretched arm, with which the LORD your God brought you out. The LORD your God will do the same to all the peoples you now fear. (Deuteronomy 7:17–19)

While they were waiting on his promises, God called them to remember what he had spoken and taught them. He reminded them how to live and love while waiting on his promises, and how they could keep themselves from forgetting.[1] God wants us to remember too, and in his grace he foresees our tendency to forget and instructs us about how to remember.

The story of the Israelites is filled with calls to remember and trust in the Lord despite the threats that surrounded them. It is a repeated call to remember the Lord's faithfulness and promises, but it is also a reminder that God never forgets his promises to us.

Alzheimer's Disease and the Second Forgetting

When we consider the story of God's people in the Old Testament, we may think the Israelites were crazy to forget and grumble. How could they forget the God who led them, rescued them, and provided for them? Why would they ever doubt a God who did such great things for them? Hadn't he promised them the land and to defeat their enemies, and didn't he then command them to take it?

When we carefully examine our own lives, we find we are not much different from the Israelites. We too have a tendency to forget, grumble, and tremble in fear. When faced with things that terrify us and push us to the brink of despair, we too forget. We forget how God has provided for us in the past and how he has promised us a brighter future, regardless of our present circumstances. We forget that God is present and lovingly caring for us, even when we are in the midst of great suffering. Sometimes we remember God's faithfulness at an intellectual level, but because our suffering is so great, we don't trust that he will be faithful again.

What threats do we face? We may not find ourselves literally wandering in the desert in search of water and food, and it is unlikely that we fear marauders as Israel did. But we know what it feels like to wander in a wilderness where we feel parched and in need of a cup of cool spiritual water. Many of us know what it feels like to face a foe that seems larger than life and impossible to defeat.

Alzheimer's can be devastating. It strikes fear, worry, and uncertainty into the hearts and minds of aging adults, their spouses, and their children. It is progressive, and there is no cure. Once

> We forget that God is present and lovingly caring for us, even when we are in the midst of great suffering.

a person develops the condition, it steadily gets worse, and nothing medical science currently offers can change the course of this brain deterioration. A person may initially forget names or appointments, but things may progress to the point that they can no longer speak, eat independently, or recognize their loving spouse or children. To argue that Alzheimer's disease is not a great threat is foolish and deceptive. It is a powerful foe.

The changes brought about by Alzheimer's can seem overwhelming. People sometimes know that things are going to get worse, and this leaves them fearful and uncertain about how soon this will happen. Others may grieve over losses they have experienced and losses that they anticipate in the future. Efforts to care for people with Alzheimer's can be filled with sadness, anger, guilt, and a range of other feelings. When we are overwhelmed by the challenges of Alzheimer's, we are prone to forget the Lord, like the Israelites in the Old Testament, and this contributes to even greater feelings of hopelessness, despair, and isolation.

The second forgetting began for Ann when her husband was diagnosed with a progressively worsening neurological condition. She knew enough about Alzheimer's to recognize that things were never going to be the same and that his condition would only get worse. Lewis was quietly terrified about what would happen next. He had always been a man of faith, and although this did not change, he had trouble focusing on God's faithfulness. Instead, he was plagued by worry for himself and his family.

When the Israelites stood on the brink of the Promised Land, they saw the enemy and were terrified. When Lewis and Ann stood at the brink of their "golden years" they were similarly terrified by the enemy of Alzheimer's disease, fearing it would defeat them and take away their lives. They may have mistakenly thought that retirement was to be their Promised Land—a place of rest—and that Alzheimer's disease had stolen this away. But this is not their true Promised Land of rest. There is more wilderness to traverse before they get there, and it cannot be stolen away. As we wander in fear and despair, we long for a cup of cool water. Even here, God calls us to trust in him, not to worry about what we will eat or drink, and to taste and see that he is good (Psalm 34:8). Soon he will bring us into the true Promised Land.

What Should We Remember?

The second forgetting reflects our tendency to forget the foundational Christian truths of:

- God's faithfulness in the past
- his presence in the midst of current trials
- his promises for the future

Although Lewis may have forgotten that he has already shared his golf story and repeated it several times throughout the day, can he remember his Lord and his story of faith? Can he remember what God has done and what he promises for Lewis's future? Similarly, can Ann remember the Lord, draw on the strength of his presence, and take comfort in his promises?

We can't do anything about the first forgetting. We cannot change the underlying damage to the brain that causes Alzheimer's. But we can address the second forgetting. We are called to help each other remember the Lord and his faithfulness regardless of our situation or the health of our brains. The command to remember God does not change, but perhaps the way we go about encouraging this does.

This is not just a book about Alzheimer's disease. It is also about how we respond to the seemingly overwhelming situations of life and the weight of suffering. How do you respond in crisis? Do you remember the Lord and look to him for help? Or do you quickly become overwhelmed to the point of panic and despair? God is not calling us to ignore the emotional and physical difficulties we face. In fact, Scripture encourages us to mourn together (Romans 12:15) and to cry out (Psalm 6). He calls us to remember him in the midst of crisis and suffering, to be still and know that he is God (Psalm 46:10). He invites us to remember all that he has done and promised. He also calls us to be present with one another in suffering, just as he is present with us. We are not called to journey through suffering alone. We need each other to help us remember.

For families in the midst of dementia care, this call to remember may seem like just one more thing you are being asked to do.

For those with dementia, this call to remember may seem like a cruel test that you think you cannot pass. After all, how can you remember God when Alzheimer's is ravaging your memory for even simple things?

For pastors and church members, it may not seem clear how you can answer the call to help people remember. (Though, as we'll see, the church is also prone to forget.)

How can any of us help each other remember the power and hope of the gospel in the midst of great trials caused by Alzheimer's disease?

As we consider these questions, never forget the wonder of the good news: God never forgets us or his promises to us, even when we forget him. Throughout Scripture, God remembers first and then acts in grace to rescue his people. Even when the Israelites forgot, God rescued them and fulfilled his promises. God's grace does not depend on what we do, including our ability to remember. Although we will suffer here on earth, God does not ultimately leave us in the brokenness of this life. He sent Christ to rescue us and to begin the process of renewal that will culminate in a new home, a promised land much better than the one Israel experienced. We can rest assured that all of this depends fully on what Christ has done for us.

We don't remember him to earn his favor or to rescue ourselves from his punishment. We remember him so that we can know a true hope in the midst of what seems hopeless. We remember him so that we can experience a peace that surpasses all understanding. We remember so that we can know how to journey with one another through the wilderness in search of our promised home — a place where there will be no tears, no suffering, and no forgetting.

FOR FURTHER REFLECTION

In this chapter we learned about the second forgetting, our tendency to forget the Lord when we are overwhelmed with the busyness and trials of this life.

- In what situations do you find yourself most prone to forget the Lord?

- What promises do you have the most trouble remembering?

- Read Deuteronomy 7:17–19. When the Israelites stood on the edge of God's Promised Land, they shook in fear because of the enemies they would face. God called them to not be afraid but to remember instead his great faithfulness in the past and to trust him that he would again deliver. What are you currently facing that feels like much more than you can manage?

- What might God be calling you to remember from the past as you face this trial? Are there specific events God is calling you to remember as evidence of how he has always been with you? How did God provide?

- How can you take courage in trusting the Lord in the present difficulty and as you face the future?

Chapter 2

UNDERSTANDING ALZHEIMER'S DISEASE

Betty gets up early each day to walk the neighborhood. She greets her neighbors, but she only uses their names about half the time; the other half of the time she avoids their names because she is unable to remember them or is afraid she will use the wrong name. The older neighbors she remembers well, but she has never been able to remember the name of the new family that moved in next door. She eats toast when she gets home and looks at the newspaper. Sometimes she reads it and sometimes she doesn't. She's seldom able to recall what she read when her husband asks her about it later. Instead, she covers this up saying, "Oh, you know, the same old thing." Her husband reminds her to take her medication after breakfast. She listens because, truth be told, she's not really sure whether she did or not. After breakfast her husband drives them to the grocery store where she helps pick out their meals for the week. She continues to do most of the cooking, although her husband is often with her while she does, double-checking to make sure she turns off the stove and oven. Later in the day her grandkids visit, and she plays card games with them and sits on the couch with them while they watch their favorite movie.

. . .

Frank has gotten lost on his drive home from his favorite coffee shop. He must have turned the wrong way when he pulled out of the parking lot but he didn't notice. He drives for a few minutes before he realizes he doesn't recognize where he is. He figures he will find his way sooner or later. For a moment he considers calling his daughter on the cell phone she bought him, but he never really figured out how to use it, so he decides to press on. He doesn't recall that this happened last month too. Although he finds his way home eventually, he isn't sure how, and his daughter is waiting for him with a worried look in her eyes. She tells him that it's time to give up driving, but since he lives alone, he can't see how that could be a good thing. This is a constant source of stress between them. Can't she see that giving up driving would mean losing his independence? His daughter is still hurt that her dad can't remember the names of her kids but is also frustrated that he seems to need more and more care. Sometimes he's up all night and sleeps during the day. He gets confused about where he put things and even believes that someone is stealing from him because he can't find his wallet and car keys.

. . .

Millie has been taking care of her husband for several years, ever since he started to lose his ability to speak. Ed had developed memory problems five years earlier, and over time he continued to decline. He lost his ability to take care of their finances. Millie had assumed he was paying the bills until the day their electricity was shut off, so she took over that responsibility. He stopped taking his medication, lost interest in getting out of the house and seeing friends, and became irritable. He would wear the same clothes several days in a row, and when she tried to tell him he only became angry and snapped at her. After he began to develop problems with speaking, things really started to get tough. He had trouble finding the words he wanted, and when he did speak, the words got so garbled that some people couldn't understand what he meant. Millie often wondered whether he was able to understand what she said to him because his replies were often confusing. Now he has trouble speaking altogether and struggles with even the most basic tasks, such as putting on clothes. He takes the shirt she hands him and rubs his hands on the material but won't put it on. He simply mumbles something she can't make out. She gently tries to put the shirt on him, but he grabs it tightly and looks at her in surprise and fear. "Get out of here! Who are you?"

• • •

Betty, Frank, and Ed are quite different people, but they share a common problem. Each has developed changes in their brains that are so small that they can only be seen under a microscope. Their impact, however, is anything but microscopic—it can often seem larger than life. Each is at a different stage of Alzheimer's disease. Betty is still in the early stages, whereas Frank and Ed are in the middle and late stages, respectively. It is important to understand these stages because they are distinct, and they help us better understand how we can care for and minister to people with Alzheimer's. If we treat a person with early-stage Alzheimer's like a person with late-stage or severe Alzheimer's, we risk insulting them by doing too much for them or oversimplifying things. Similarly, if we treat a person with severe, late-stage Alzheimer's like a person with mild dementia, we will frustrate them, put their safety at risk, and be unable to reach them effectively.

Although Alzheimer's is one of the most devastating and feared conditions among older people, it can develop, in rare instances, in people in their thirties and forties. As many as 30 to 40 percent of people in their eighties have this dreaded disease. Alzheimer's has grown increasingly common over the past several decades as advances in medical technology and care have enabled people to live longer. As many as one in seven adults over the age of seventy-one is affected by the condition, and the number of people with Alzheimer's may triple by the year 2050.[1] Healthcare spending on Alzheimer's disease and dementia is currently greater than what is spent on cancer and heart disease combined.

Although millions of dollars are spent on Alzheimer's research each year, we still do not have a good understanding of what causes it, and sadly we do not have a cure. Although much is unknown, we have learned quite a bit as well. This chapter addresses common questions.

What Is Alzheimer's Disease?

The human brain is beautiful and complex, delicate yet resilient. Humans have 100 billion neurons (brain cells) that are connected to each other in a network that communicates within the brain and to other parts of the body. Neurons are incredibly small (4–18 microns or 0.0004 to 0.0018 centimeters) and communicate with each other via chemicals that pass from one cell to another in a coordinated network of connections throughout the brain. When this brain activity occurs, there is a resulting response such as a physical movement, speech, or recollection of a memory. While you are reading this, the neurons in your brain are communicating with each other via these chemical transmissions. It happens seamlessly so that you don't notice it until something goes wrong. The fascinating complexity and efficiency of the brain should prompt us to glorify God along with the psalmist for the beauty of his creation:

> *For you created my inmost being;*
> *you knit me together in my mother's womb.*
> *I praise you because I am fearfully and wonderfully made;*
> *your works are wonderful,*
> *I know that full well.*

> (PSALM 139:13–14)

But something has gone wrong. For reasons we do not yet know, a series of changes take place in brains that develop Alzheimer's disease. This begins when naturally occurring substances (certain proteins) in the brain begin to act in an abnormal fashion. This sets in motion a cascade of changes leading to progressive brain damage. Eventually we notice changes in the person and begin to forget the beauty of the brain. We once again experience living in a broken world.

If you have Alzheimer's disease, here is what likely happened:[2] Something known as amyloid precursor protein exists on the outside of neurons (one type of cells in your brain), and it helps to maintain healthy brain functioning. At some point, an enzyme encounters this amyloid precursor protein and snips it into fragments, which then clump together into sticky deposits, called plaques, which disrupt the communication between the neurons. This is the earliest change we see in the brains of people with Alzheimer's.

Each neuron has an internal support system that helps the neuron stay healthy. Microtubules are part of this support system. They are akin to a set of train tracks that transport nutrients within the neuron. *Tau* is a protein that is embedded within these tracks, and for unknown reasons it breaks off in brains with Alzheimer's and form into tangles. The microtubules disintegrate and can no longer transport nutrients, leading to cell death.

Plaques and tangles are followed by damage and shrinkage, also known as atrophy, of brain tissue. A certain amount of brain shrinkage is normal. As people get older, their brain tissue shrinks a bit, but there is little obvious effect on thinking and memory. Brains with Alzheimer's disease experience much greater shrinkage (Figure 1).

These changes begin gradually, and often people don't notice the changes in their thinking or behavior until much later. In fact, scientists have discovered that the plaques and tangles may begin as early as ten to twenty years *before* the first memory problems that the person and their family notice (often referred to as "preclinical Alzheimer's").[3] Eventually, the changes become severe enough that memory gets noticeably worse.

The plaques and tangles typically start in areas of the brain known as the temporal lobes, which are on the sides of the brain near the ears. The hippocampus is a part of the temporal lobes, and it converts short-term memory to long-term memory. Alzheimer's damages the hippocampus (Figure 2), which is why the earliest

> The longer the person lives with the disease, the more severe and widespread the underlying brain changes will become. As these changes spread, they begin to overwhelm the person, and as the person is overwhelmed, so is their family.

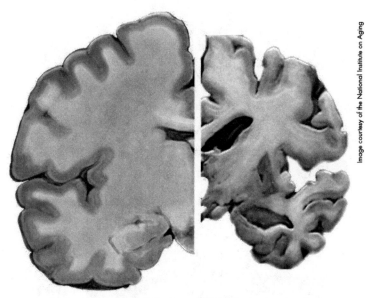

Image courtesy of the National Institute on Aging

Figure 1 Cross sections of a healthy brain (left) and a brain severely damaged by Alzheimer's disease in the late stages. Note the significant shrinkage (atrophy) of brain tissue due to Alzheimer's disease.

and most noticeable symptom of Alzheimer's is difficulty recalling recent information.

As in Betty's case, these changes develop slowly, and at first they are not severe enough to interfere with memory or daily functioning. As they continue to accumulate, they damage more brain tissue and disrupt communication between brain cells, which over time interferes with memory. Because this accumulation of plaques and tangles happens slowly over time, the development of memory loss and other changes in functioning is quite subtle at first, making it hard for people to determine whether a given instance of memory failure represents normal aging or something more serious.

Unfortunately, as time goes on, the plaques and tangles spread from the hippocampus and temporal lobes to other parts of the brain, including the parietal and frontal lobes (Figure 2). As a result, other aspects of functioning are impacted (as in the cases of Frank and Ed). Alzheimer's is *progressive*—the longer the person lives with the

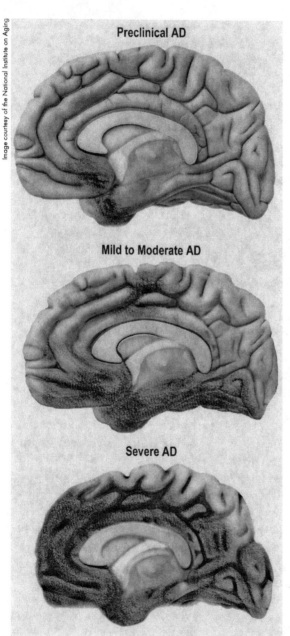

Preclinical AD

Mild to Moderate AD

Severe AD

Image courtesy of the National Institute on Aging

Figure 2 Cross sections of three brains with Alzheimer's pathology. These images represent, from top to bottom, the brains of people with preclinical to mild (Betty), mild to moderate (Frank), and severe (Ed) Alzheimer's disease.

disease, the more severe and widespread the underlying brain changes will become. As these changes spread, they begin to overwhelm the person, and as the person is overwhelmed, so is their family.

How Is Alzheimer's Diagnosed?

You might be surprised to learn that even though the plaques and tangles are the underlying problem, the diagnosis of Alzheimer's disease does not rely on the detection of these plaques and tangles. Typical brain scans (MRIs or CTs, for example) cannot detect them because they are too small. The only way to identify plaques and tangles is with an autopsy of the brain—after the person has died. Instead, making a diagnosis of Alzheimer's disease focuses on loss of memory and other cognitive changes and ruling out other medical causes of those changes. When you report memory changes to your doctors, they may give you a screening test to help determine whether you are having cognitive problems apart from those brought about by normal aging. The screening tests take a few minutes. They may ask you to remember a few words or to draw something.

Through a medical exam, lab tests (such as a blood test), and a brain scan, they will attempt to identify potential causes of these changes. A brain scan may be used to rule out other causes such as a stroke, brain tumor, or reversible conditions like hydrocephalus (sometimes known as "water on the brain"). Emerging technologies that utilize advanced imaging (PET with amyloid imaging) can now demonstrate the presence of plaques in the brain while the person is still living, but currently this is not a part of typical diagnostic procedures. It is still an experimental research procedure only offered at specialized centers. Even with this new technology, it is likely that diagnosis will continue to involve two pieces: (1) evaluation of memory and other areas of cognitive change and (2) consideration of the potential causes of these changes. As other causes are ruled out, the diagnosis of Alzheimer's becomes more likely. This is particularly true when the primary changes involve a gradual onset of memory problems and then progressive worsening over time.

Is There a Cure?

When people are diagnosed with a major medical conditions like cancer or heart disease, they are quick to inquire about medical treatment. If you have an infection you will receive antibiotics, and things quickly improve. Even for more chronic conditions like high blood pressure and diabetes, there are lifestyle changes that a person can make, in addition to medication, that lead to restoration of health. We live in an age of amazing medical advancements, and we have come to expect effective treatments for every acute and chronic medical condition. This is why, when people are diagnosed with Alzheimer's and other dementias, they are quick to think of it as they would any other medical condition — an infection, high blood pressure, diabetes, or cancer.

But Alzheimer's is different. There is no cure, and most scientists admit that they are not even sure what *causes* the changes (the plaques and tangles) in the first place. Hopefully a cure will be discovered at some point, but various groups have estimated that without a major scientific breakthrough, this will not happen for many years. When we say that we cannot cure Alzheimer's disease, we mean that we cannot rid the person of the underlying brain changes and symptoms. Experimental treatments are focusing on removal of amyloid plaques, and these appear promising in preliminary studies. They can remove the plaques in rats and mice, but memory and learning are not improved. Effective treatments for human beings are still a long way off. This means that if you currently have Alzheimer's, it is unlikely that any of these experimental treatments will noticeably benefit your memory, but you can pray that they will benefit future generations.[4]

What Medical Treatment Is Available?

Although medicine currently cannot halt the progress of plaques and tangles, several medications may help reduce the cognitive symptoms. Earlier I mentioned that Alzheimer's disrupts the normal chemical communication between brain cells (neurons). A chemical called *acetylcholine* was originally thought to be the primary neurochemical disrupted in Alzheimer's disease, and most existing medical treatments for Alzheimer's seek to enhance memory by boosting levels of this chemical. The effectiveness of these medicines is somewhat controversial, although the research is clear on several points. These medicines do not *reverse* cognitive symptoms or return memory to normal levels. They also do not impact the underlying plaques and tangles (they weren't designed to do this). Some patients and families may report benefits of these treatments, and this is important. Long-term studies, however, do not show a significant difference between treated and untreated people with Alzheimer's in terms of their cognitive functioning. Even the best treatments seem to have minimal impact on memory problems over the long term.[5] Another class of medications known as *memantine* works in a similar fashion but is designed to affect a different aspect of brain chemistry. This may be offered by your doctor in combination with the medicines that affect acetylcholine.

You can certainly ask your doctor about these medicines, and they are worth considering. But it is important to understand what these medicines will and will not do. In the best-case scenarios, these medicines *may* help maintain cognitive functioning for a period of time, which will give you more time and delay your need for greater assistance. But these changes may be difficult to notice. It isn't likely that you will notice immediate changes if you take these medications. The underlying disease will continue to progress and worsen. In other words, the hope offered by current medicines is minimal — although there are still good reasons to ask your doctor about them. But be aware that even those who respond well to the current, approved medications will eventually show further decline in their memory and functioning.

What Can I Expect?

The bad news is that Alzheimer's disease will continue to get worse. Because it's a progressive disease, meaning that the underlying changes spread and inflict further brain decay, it is inevitable that this will affect more and more of a person's thinking and behavior.

In the earliest stages, the changes may be so mild that it is difficult to determine whether they are just normal "senior moments" or something worse. These can include struggling to find the right word, forgetting where a purse or car keys were left, or forgetting the names of new people. All of these symptoms can also happen with normal aging. Eventually a person moves into a stage where they have more difficulty with instrumental activities of daily living: paying bills, managing a checkbook, cooking a complex recipe, or planning a project.

As time passes, confusion about the day, time, or even the season can set in. It is relatively common for people to think they are younger and live as if it were twenty years ago or think that they are living in their old house (even when they live in an assisted-living facility). They may become confused about their personal information and aspects of their life history.

Eventually a person may progress to a stage in which he or she may forget the names of close family members, including their spouse or children. In more severe stages, assistance with basic activities of living such as dressing, eating, or using the bathroom might become necessary. In the latest stages the ability to speak, comprehend, and walk can be lost, although not all individuals reach this stage.

Many people, though not all, will develop behavior problems. These can occur in different types of dementia and across various stages, but they become more common as dementia progresses. These problems include wandering, agitation, depression, anxiety, irritability, problems with sleep, delusions (believing things that are obviously untrue — "people are stealing from me"), hallucinations (seeing or hearing things that aren't there), and disinhibition (loss of behavioral control).

The stages in this chart should be used to help think about the differences

> In the earliest stages, the changes may be so mild that it is difficult to determine whether they are just normal "senior moments" or something worse.

	Stage		
	Early/Mild	Middle/Moderate	Late/Severe
Person	Betty	Frank	Ed
Examples of changes	Memory problems begin	Confusion about time and date	Needs help with personal care
	Difficulty finding right words	Getting lost in familiar places	May not speak often and difficult to understand
	Trouble with some everyday tasks such as managing money or medication	Wandering	Difficulty with walking and swallowing
	Trouble planning and anticipating consequences	Trouble picking appropriate clothing	Difficulty recognizing faces

between people in early, middle, and late stages of the disease, but caution should be used in projecting what a person will experience in the future. These stages overlap in terms of the symptoms and problems experienced. Each individual with Alzheimer's progresses at a different rate, and no one can predict how quickly or to what extent they will progress.[6]

The progressive, untreatable nature of dementia creates considerable fear and uncertainty for people with dementia and their families.[7] People experience uncertainty about their condition and their future. Those with dementia (and their families) have uncertainty about what additional changes will come as the disease progresses and when these changes will occur. People with dementia may wonder if they will eventually lose the ability to recognize their loved ones or if they will lose their most cherished memories. Some of the things people hold most dear may be lost, and this can be understandably painful and terrifying.

At this point, we do not have much hope that we can halt these cognitive changes. If you or a loved one have Alzheimer's disease, this is certainly discouraging news. Most likely you started out with some hope that medicine would change this situation. But I don't want to leave you hopeless. Please keep reading, because we are not without hope. Yes, there is suffering to come, but the reality of suffering does not take away our hope.

Living with Alzheimer's

Even though the outlook is not positive for treating Alzheimer's disease, we are not without hope and we are never alone. We need to learn how to lean on, trust in, and remember our Lord and the powerful promises of the gospel in the midst of the Alzheimer's disease journey. It can be tempting to believe that the future holds nothing but decay and deterioration, followed by death. Reading about the lack of effective treatments may leave you feeling overwhelmed, not sure what the future holds. Alzheimer's is a problem that is bigger than we are and more than we can face alone. And like the Israelites, we can see what we are up against and quickly grow discouraged. We forget where our foundation lies, where our future hope is placed. At times like this, we may feel like God's people did in Deuteronomy 7:17: "You may say to yourselves, 'These nations are stronger than we are. How can we drive them out?'"

Learning about Alzheimer's disease leaves people fearful. Alzheimer's is a formidable foe. Much like the ten spies who reported to Moses that they could never defeat the people living in the land, we are tempted to give up and admit defeat. But God has another word for us to hear. He wants us to turn our eyes away from our enemy, Alzheimer's, and to focus on him. He wants us to remember his powerful and wonderful acts, and his amazing promises for our future: "Do not be terrified by them, for the LORD your God, who is among you, is a great and awesome God" (7:21).

Alzheimer's is terrifying. That is true. But the greater truth is that God is with us, and he has defeated our enemy—even the devastating power of Alzheimer's. To experience this victory, we need to have a battle strategy. We need to learn how to remember God, even as memories are lost and our bodies fail and falter. God is calling us to redirect our attention from the bad news of Alzheimer's to the good news of hope in the gospel of Jesus Christ.

. . . .

FOR FURTHER REFLECTION

In this chapter we learned some of the basics of Alzheimer's disease, one of the most feared and dreaded conditions of later life.

- If you have Alzheimer's disease, take some time to talk with a loved one about what is most difficult about having Alzheimer's.

- If you don't have Alzheimer's, consider what you've learned in this chapter and discuss what you think would be the hardest part of living with this disease. Why is it so terrifying to so many people?

. . . .

Chapter 3

REMEMBERING AND FORGETTING

MEMORY IS FILLED WITH MYSTERY. Some of our memories are beautiful; some are tragic and sad. Memories can make us feel happy and comfortable, or they can trigger pain and shame. Our memory systems are beautiful in their elegance and complexity, but they are frustrated and fallen, like everything else in this world. Sometimes it's a struggle just to remember the everyday details of life — what we have to do and where we need to go. We forget things more often than we like to admit.

● ● ●

When Charles woke up this morning, he felt groggy and unusually tired. He looked around and was immediately confused. This wasn't his home. The pictures on the nightstand were familiar, but his wife wasn't next to him in bed. A familiar voice called his name, and a nurse walked into his room to tell him it was time for breakfast.

Now, his grown children and his wife are visiting him, but he can't always remember their names. He shows them recognition and affection in his hugs and is glad to see them. He calls his wife by her name about half the time, and each time she feels a small sense of relief. He doesn't always understand that he is living in a nursing home. Sometimes he thinks it is a poorly run hotel. Earlier, he complained loudly to the staff that he hadn't had his breakfast. But the drops of syrup on his shirt suggest otherwise. Each day the nursing staff tries to orient him by telling him the day of the week, the date, the year, and the season. His forgetting causes confusion, and in his fear and uncertainty, he sometimes lashes out at those who try to care for him.

Charles can talk at length about his work as an engineer. Sometimes his explanations are confusing, but at other times his accounts are interesting and informative. He tells stories about when his children were young, repeating anecdotes several times in a two-hour span. When someone reads a favorite psalm, he quickly joins in, reciting each cherished word. When he hears an old hymn, he raises his hands slowly and breathes each word quietly, his face reflecting a peace that surpasses understanding. As the song continues, he sings more audibly, with joy and enthusiasm—seeming more alive than he has been in weeks.

Yet as the day drags on, he becomes confused again and wants to go home. In fact, he often demands to go home, not understanding why the people in charge won't help him get there. After the family leaves, he shouts at one of his favorite nurses, who gently redirects him to his room, where she turns on his old radio. He soon settles down to listen to the news. He falls asleep, unaware that he will not remember any of these events tomorrow.

Charles lives in the fog of dementia. Although there is much he cannot remember, there are some things that he *can* remember—despite the changes that Alzheimer's has wrought on his brain. On the surface, it doesn't seem to make sense. How can he remember things that happened thirty years ago, while forgetting that he ate breakfast? How does he remember the words of a cherished song better than the day or date?

As you and I go about our day, we constantly form new memories, some of which we will recall later, some others we will not. Think about your day right now. What have you done? What do you have left to do? You may recall taking a shower before getting dressed. You probably remember whether you ate breakfast. You make mental checklists and check off the items you needed to accomplish. You can remember if your spouse asked you to pick up milk on your drive home. You can remember your boss asking if you would be willing to take on new responsibilities. You might even remember that today is your wife's birthday.

Your brain stores tasks, events, and conversations for later recall. Without Alzheimer's, your brain is beautifully efficient. Most of the time you don't need to think about any of this. When you do forget something, a gentle reminder is all you need.

But the brain of a person with Alzheimer's has great difficulty storing new memories and recalling them later. Imagine, for a moment, that you are no longer certain if you ate breakfast or whether you took a shower this morning. Without a clear memory, you might look for signs to help you figure these things out. You try to notice if you feel hungry, or if you smell like soap, or if you have wet hair. These cues help you to figure out whether these events have happened or not. Sometimes this works, but at other times it fails, and you simply have no memory of an event or a conversation. Unless you write it down, you will not remember that your spouse asked you to buy milk. Because your brain did not store the memory, you might even be quite certain that it did *not* happen, and you may start arguing with someone about it. Even if you do write it down, you may not remember doing it, and you are confused by the reminder. You may grow suspicious of others because they are trying to convince you of things that you simply cannot remember.

Or imagine this. As you read this book, a friend stops by and asks you why you are reading it — *again*. You are confused and tell him that you are only partway through and haven't finished it yet. In response, he gives you a puzzled look and tells you that you read the whole book and discussed it with him last week. You try to correct him, certain this did not happen, but your friend is adamant — you have already read this book! You grow frustrated, perhaps even angry.

As you can see, living with memory problems is more than a little disconcerting.

Memory Routes

There are different routes into a person's memory. These follow paths, or connections, between brain cells, and these paths are formed through our experiences over our lifetime. Although human brains are fairly uniform in their structure, these microlevel connections are unique to each individual and are tied to what they've experienced. Within any human brain, certain regions and pathways play key roles in different aspects of memory. Alzheimer's disease damages some of these regions and connections, while others are relatively spared.

When we begin to explore a person's memory, we may go back to an earlier time of life when they were younger and healthier. We might ask them how they felt in different situations as they recall past life events. Memory includes the unconscious aspects of life as well, movements or actions that are carried out regularly and consistently with little thought or conscious intention. The oft-quoted saying "It's like riding a bike" refers to these unconscious aspects of memory. You don't have to think about them, and you don't quickly forget them.

In this chapter we will look at the different types of memory and to what extent these are affected by Alzheimer's. One of the goals in treating those with Alzheimer's is to improve their ability to remember. Attempts have been made to do this through medication, using crossword puzzles, and even dietary changes. But most of these attempts focus on a specific aspect of memory, paying relatively little attention to other aspects. Memory is more than just the recollection of facts or events; it also involves things we feel and do and, to some extent, less conscious aspects of who we are.

So before we look at ways of improving memory, we need to ask: What, exactly, are we trying to remember? It can certainly be helpful to remember whether you ate breakfast or where you stashed your money. But it's quite another thing to remember who you are and what your life history is — the people you are related to and

> Memory is more than just the recollection of facts or events; it also involves things we feel and do and, to some extent, less conscious aspects of who we are.

where you lived, for example. When we begin to experience the challenges of Alzheimer's, what we need is not just a memory intervention or some helpful techniques, we need a whole new way of *living* with the reality of pervasive memory failure.

What Should We Remember?

What should we remember? Consider several examples below. How important would you say it is to remember

- to take your medication
- how to get to a friend's home
- the name of a new neighbor or grandchild
- where you put your purse or wallet

Each of these draws upon a particular form of memory that is affected in early Alzheimer's. Unless you have the disease, or know someone who does, you probably don't think about having to remember these things. Most of the time you remember them naturally and without effort. The ability of the brain to store and retrieve information is impressive, and it reflects a design with exquisite detail. It is nothing short of a miracle that we remember anything, but the sheer number of things we remember is truly staggering. The process the brain uses to store a memory involves a variety of brain circuits, neurochemicals, and new connections that are formed between neurons. The efficiency of this system is amazing. It should cause us to stop and give praise to God for his magnificent design!

Although God's creation is beautiful when it functions as intended, we live in a world where things don't always function that way. The Bible tells us that the world we live in is fallen, broken by human sin and rebellion, a world filled with disorder and decay (Genesis 3; Romans 8:18–23). All of creation has been impacted, including the spiritual and physical. This affects our brains in such a way that we are prone to two forms of forgetting in particular—neurological memory impairment due to Alzheimer's disease, and the forgetting of the Lord due to spiritual memory impairment.

Remembering—who God is, who we are, and what our purpose is in this world—is one of God's primary commands for us. But because we live in a fallen world, we struggle to do this.

> When people develop Alzheimer's they do not forget everything — they still retain some key memories.

Growing old brings expectations of accumulated wisdom and honor. But not everyone experiences that. In fact, many experience a dramatic forgetting instead, an experience that erodes the blessing of growing old with honor and hinders passing along the wisdom that has been gained over a lifetime. This is tragic.

Yet we need to hear that God provides grace to us, even in our forgetting. When people develop Alzheimer's they do not forget everything—they still retain some key memories. These are arguably more important than the "daily detail" memories we rely upon for everyday conversations and events. But God's grace is still present, even when these details are forgotten. Let's look a bit more deeply at how God's grace works through the way he designed our memory. Consider how we can draw upon the memory that is spared from the initial effects of dementia to fully live our life before God (John 10:10).

Where Remembering Is Most Difficult

Decades of research have demonstrated that there are multiple memory systems in the brain. We will consider three of them.[1] The differences between these memory systems have implications for how we help people with Alzheimer's disease as they try to remember their own life story and their faith in God.

The first (and most difficult) form of memory for people with Alzheimer's is consciously recalling events or conversations that happened in the recent past (known as declarative memory). This memory system and its underlying brain structures are typically the first to be affected. The plaques and tangles damage the hippocampus and nearby brain structures, and this prevents people from storing new information into long-term memory. If you ask them about yesterday or even earlier today, they may not remember. They may try to cover this up or deflect the question, but in all likelihood this information is simply not there for them.

Obviously, this is a key cause of difficulty for people with Alzheimer's and their families. People cannot remember if they took their medication, paid their bills, put something on the stove, or turned it off. In some cases, they cannot remember where they were going when they left the house. Much has been written about what people with Alzheimer's *cannot* do, but instead of focusing on these details, let's explore what people with Alzheimer's *can* do and remember.

What Can Those with Alzheimer's Remember?

Remembering the Distant Past

"Why can my mother remember what happened thirty years ago but not this morning?" This is one of the first and most common questions I get from families struggling to deal with the changes wrought by Alzheimer's and dementia. It's baffling that a person can remember the details of events that happened decades ago but has very little memory of things that happened last week, yesterday, or even earlier today. Normally, we expect a person to recall recent events better than those from the distant past. Yet in Alzheimer's disease, the opposite is true. The memory of recent events is disrupted, while older memories seem to be preserved.

In truth, the older memories are not as good as they once were, but they are less affected by the disease than recent ones. Memory is complex, but the explanation is actually quite simple. Because the initial damage is to the temporal lobes, an area of the brain involved in storage of memory, these recent memories are not effectively stored. For the person, it's as if the events never happened.

Older memories stick around, however. They were stored long before the onset of Alzheimer's and remain available for later recall. So although people with the disease have trouble storing new information, they can still access older information that was effectively stored before the disease began to ravage their brains.[2]

In addition, these older memories have been rehearsed and retold many times, making them more accessible. Sometimes people rehearse them out loud by telling stories to others, while at other times the rehearsal is in the person's mind during moments of solitude. These older memories are often quite meaningful to them, filled with great joy or sorrow. In helping people with Alzheimer's remember, we must first begin to build upon these older, autobiographical memories.

Remembering Actions

In addition to memories of the past, we have a procedural memory system. This system helps us remember how to perform certain actions without having to think about them. These are the memories that—as stated before—are like "riding a bike." When you see a bike, you probably walk toward it and without thinking about it can get on and start pedaling. You don't need to stop and think, "Hmm … what do I do first here?"

Procedural memories can come back to a person even when they can't remember having done the action before. A person may even doubt that they know how to perform the action because they can't remember doing it recently. An HBO series called *The Alzheimer's Project*[3] follows Woody, a man who has been living with symptoms of Alzheimer's for over a decade. Woody is unable to remember what people have told him after a few minutes or to find his way around the facility where he lives. Before developing dementia, he was an accomplished singer who participated in an a cappella group. In the documentary, his wife and daughter pick him up and take him to a concert by the group he sang with in the past. On the way he asks where they are going every minute or two. His memory is clearly impaired. When told that he will be singing, he is doubtful. Soon after arriving, they bring him on stage with the rest of the group, and a few seconds after the group starts singing, he immediately joins in and leads with a solo—never missing a word. On the drive back, he has no memory that this occurred.

Procedural memory is less affected by Alzheimer's disease because it is less reliant upon the temporal lobes and the hippocampus.

Instead, this system is tied to other brain structures (called the *caudate nuclei*) that lie deeper within the brain and influence the formation of habits and physical movements. This doesn't mean that people with Alzheimer's can still do *all* of the physical activities they once did. The reality is that there will be changes here too, but I mention this as one avenue because we can use it to help people remember and practice their faith. The procedural memory system provides a different route for remembering God and practicing faith. It can provide some level of meaning and assurance, even in the midst of the confusion that results from the loss of memories. As people become more disconnected over time, this memory system provides anchors for their identity.

Remembering Emotional Events

Emotional memory is the third memory system. These memories rely on a brain structure called the *amygdala*. This form of memory involves remembering events that had strong emotions attached to them. Emotional memory is also about remembering how you felt in certain situations. You experience this aspect of memory when you visit places where something significant happened to you, whether good or bad. The sights, smells, and sounds bring back feelings that you might not consciously recall. You don't consciously think, "Now what was that like back then? How did I feel?" The feeling comes back before you consciously recall the details of the experience.

Some research suggests that people can remember emotional aspects of memory even when they can't remember what happened. The resilience of our emotional memory system was beautifully displayed in a study of people who have amnesia due to damage to their hippocampus.[4] These people were asked to watch short film clips designed to prompt positive and negative emotions. A short time after they watched the clips, they were largely unable to recall details of any clip, but they were able to recall how it made them feel, even if they didn't know why.[5]

As we have seen, both procedural and emotional memories are stronger in people with Alzheimer's than their memories of recent facts, events, and people. These forms of memory can influence emotion, thought, and behavior in the absence of conscious recollection or even the intention to remember.[6] In other words, some memories influence our lives and are displayed in how we behave and live—even when we cannot consciously recall them.

Why Does This Matter?

Think about the different ways you interact with people. When I get home from work, the first thing I do is ask questions: How was your day? What did you do? Do you remember that we're having dinner with our friends tonight?

Obviously, this doesn't work for people with Alzheimer's. Such questions draw heavily on the memory system that is most impaired. Though these questions seem simple, they highlight the person's memory deficits. Instead of asking such questions, we should try to interact in a way that draws upon their life story (older memories), their well-worn behavioral patterns (procedural memories), and those aspects of life that are flavored with emotion. This will draw upon their "memory strengths."

These interactions also provide the person with anchors. Despite their confusion about the present, people can continue to find themselves and reconnect to their faith by rehearsing their story with people who love and care for them. Sometimes younger people are frustrated when older people with memory impairments talk more about the past than the present. Now, hopefully, you understand why they do this. The truth is that we all prefer to talk about things we know well rather than things of which we are uncertain. Reminiscing about the past is important for those who are confused or even upset about the present. It supports positive emotions, is a mechanism for connecting and drawing closer to other people, and helps them to stay rooted in the things and events that have helped define them.

These older, personal memories also draw upon emotional memory and are typically formed before the onset of significant damage to the brain. As the disease advances, the details of these events may still be affected, but the ability to recall them in some form, with the help of a loved one, remains an island of grace as the flood waters of disease threaten to overwhelm the person.

The work of remembering can be done with family and friends. Sometimes there may be inaccuracies or mistakes, but as long as they are not harmful, these can be overlooked. The listener should remember that this is not a quiz; it is a chance to connect, honor, and love the person. Active listening shows love and honor to the person remembering.

With the help of loving family and friends, people with Alzheimer's disease can remain connected with their story—including their journey of faith—and this can prompt a deeper remembering for them. A person may recall the words to an old song of faith or how to take Communion or how to recite the Lord's Prayer. When this happens, we may marvel that the person is still quite capable in this regard. One of the temptations of caregivers is to assume that memory is uniformly impaired. We can thank our God that even though the world and our brains are broken, his grace has spared certain memory systems that continue to allow us to connect with him in unique ways. In a parched land of forgetting, this is a cup of cool water that we can cherish, if even for just a few brief moments.

Decay and Grace in Memory

While we pray and hope that methods to undo or prevent the damage caused by Alzheimer's will eventually be developed, we can also ask the Lord to show us how to live life to the fullest even with Alzheimer's disease. Christians profess that their hope is in Christ, and we believe that Christ came so that we might have abundant life (John 10:10). We have hope for the next life—and that is wonderful. But God is also concerned with the way we live right now. He wants us to have hope in him in this life as well.

If you are struggling with the early stages of Alzheimer's disease, it might feel as though you are mired in despair. Much has been lost, and you can't help but mourn what is likely to be lost in the future. But God calls us to turn our eyes toward him. Psalm 121:1–8 says:

I lift up my eyes to the mountains—
*   where does my help come from?*
My help comes from the LORD,
*   the Maker of heaven and earth.*

He will not let your foot slip—
*   he who watches over you will not slumber;*
indeed, he who watches over Israel
*   will neither slumber nor sleep.*

The LORD watches over you—
*   the LORD is your shade at your right hand;*
the sun will not harm you by day,
*   nor the moon by night.*

The LORD will keep you from all harm—
*   he will watch over your life;*
the LORD will watch over your coming and going
*   both now and forevermore.*

Our hope comes from a God who is stronger than Alzheimer's. When we face the confusion and uncertainty of this disease, God calls us to remember him, and in his grace he provides us the ability to do so.

A woman was referred to me for memory testing. I asked her to share her daily routine with me. She lived in an assisted-living facility, and each morning she would get up early and walk to the chapel, where she would sit and pray to God. She took great comfort in this, and that time with the Lord was clearly meaningful to her. As we began to test her memory, it was obvious to both of us that she was struggling. As a professional, I could see that Alzheimer's disease was the likely diagnosis.

We never finished her testing, however, because at one point she promptly quit. I asked her why, and she told me that even though her memory didn't look good on the test, it was "just fine for what I do." And she was right. She took time each day to pray and spend time with the Lord, and this was the most important part of her day. Even though her memory impairment meant that she sometimes got lost on her way back from praying, her memory of the Lord brought her back each day.

Even as our bodies decay and fail us, God's grace enables us to remember what is truly important. We live between the already and the not-yet, leaning on the unshakeable truth that we are already redeemed in Christ but have not yet been fully restored. Our memories fail, and it is in these moments that we fall most heavily upon God's grace, his remembrance of us.

> Each morning she would get up early and walk to the chapel, where she would sit and pray to God. . . . Her memory of the Lord brought her back each day.

If you are struggling with hopelessness right now, let me encourage you to jump ahead to the last chapter. It's okay. We need reminders of these things when we struggle, and that's one of the reasons I've written this book. The truth that I want you to hear is that no matter how much we may forget, even if we forget him—God will never forget us.

Repeat this to yourself each day. Write it down. Ask a friend to remind you of this truth:

No matter what happens to you, God cannot and will not forget you.

Remember this for your own comfort, but know that if you forget to remember, he will not.

FOR FURTHER REFLECTION

In this chapter we learned that memory is more than the recollection of facts and recent events. Memories involving actions, emotions, and the distant past can influence our life in the present, even though we may not be aware of them.

- How will this influence the way you interact with someone who has Alzheimer's? How can you use the broader understanding of memory to help them remember the Lord?

- If you aren't involved in Alzheimer's care, how can you use this to better remember the Lord in the busyness of daily life?

Chapter 4

THE GOSPEL FOR THOSE WITH ALZHEIMER'S

Henry was a missionary in Asia for years. He was a faithful member of his church, and he has been a loving father and husband for over fifty years. He loves the Lord and God's Word. When he began forgetting things, it was difficult to know if it was just a normal part of aging, poor hearing, or something else. Unfortunately, any uncertainty disappeared over time as he began to forget to pay the bills and how to use certain household tools. Eventually, he had trouble remembering and recognizing his grandchildren. Now, he is no longer able to help around the house or yard. In fact, he needs to be helped with the basic activities of daily living. It is difficult for him to speak, and when he does, he still seems withdrawn. When he's awake, he stares straight ahead, saying little unless directly spoken to.

Once, his memory troubles frustrated him. He would hit his hand on his head to jar his brain into remembering. Now, it's hard to tell when he's frustrated because he says so little. This once brilliant man, known for his way with words and his critical analysis of difficult problems, has been reduced to silence, a silence broken by groans of pain and frustration.

People live anywhere from three to twenty years after being diagnosed with dementias like Alzheimer's disease. Most average about six to twelve years. What is life like during this time? People are terrified of dementia because we tend to only hear about the decline and decay that leads to death. We are tempted to believe that people with dementia have no hope because there is no cure for Alzheimer's and treatments are lacking. The progressive loss of memory leads people to believe that they will become unreachable and unknowable. Intentionally or not, many tend to believe that because people with dementia cannot contribute (in work, around the house, at church), they have little or no value. No hope, no identity, and no value—is it any surprise to hear that people dread Alzheimer's disease more than any other medical condition?[1] Is there more to dementia than this depressing storyline?

The stories we tell inform our lives and influence the way we think about difficulty and struggle. Our stories also inform the way we treat those who live and die with Alzheimer's.[2] So is there a storyline that helps us understand dementia? What does the biblical story have to say about this disease? What relevance does God's Word have to this experience?

The Bible tells us that God has a definite storyline for us to live by, one that we often fail to recognize or remember. God's story transforms our individual stories, giving them new meaning, even when they involve suffering. God's story forces us to reconsider our expectations, where we have settled into acceptance and where we have doubted or lost hope. In the midst of this, we meet God, who is described as one "who is able to do immeasurably more than all we ask or imagine, according to his power that is at work within us" (Ephesians 3:20).

I have found that the story of the Bible provides us with a way to understand the individual stories and experiences of people with Alzheimer's. In particular, four themes from the broader biblical story apply: creation, fall, redemption, and restoration. Understanding these themes is an important step toward understanding Alzheimer's disease. Why? Because these four themes unfold a narrative of hope, and they answer the core questions that lie at the heart of living, suffering, and dying with this condition:

- Who am I? How do I understand and maintain identity in suffering and decline?
- Where can I find hope in the midst of Alzheimer's? Hope for living in the present? Hope in the face of death?

Identity: Who Am I?

The biblical story opens by telling us that we were created by a loving God for two purposes:

- To live with him and to honor and glorify him in our everyday life.
- To live in community with other people, loving them and serving them, and, by doing this, loving our Creator with our whole life.

We were created to give God glory. We are the pinnacle of his creation, specifically created in his image. Our beginnings display a magnificent design, and we continue to see this when we delve deeply into brain structure and function. The complexity and beauty of the human body and brain are magnificent and bring glory to God, our Creator. We were meant to be a glorious creation, reflecting God's image and goodness — more beautiful than the best sunset. More intricately designed than the microchip that powers your smartphone. More intelligent and powerful than any creature on the planet. Our creation helps answer the questions of who are we, where we came from, and what we were designed to do.

Living beneath the weight of Alzheimer's, this may seem like a nice story — a fairy tale disconnected from your daily reality. If you are taking care of someone who is advancing through the stages of dementia, you may not be rejoicing over the beauty of the brain.

This is so because sin entered into the story and led to disastrous consequences. Every aspect of creation is affected. Not only did sin and disobedience affect our relationship with God, they also led to brokenness throughout creation. We all, without exception, experience frustration, decay, and death. The story of the fall and the reality of human sin and rebellion against our Creator recognizes that there are now great difficulties in life (Genesis 3). Although there was once a time when Adam and Eve walked with God and there was no suffering, we now experience a separation from God and suffering is part of the fabric of life.[3]

We see these effects in dementia. The brain doesn't work right, and you can't just snap out of it by trying harder. Real damage has been done to the brain. Many caregivers have shared that they feel as if they are losing the person to a kind of living death. As the plaques and tangles contribute to brain decay, the person seems to decay as well, leaving many caregivers feeling hopeless and depleted. The fall makes sense of all this in that in their rebellion, Adam and Eve "died spiritually, and their bodies also began to experience gradual decay that ultimately led to their physical deaths,"[4] and this was passed along to the rest of humanity.[5] The beautiful creation was no longer as it was created to be — suffering and death entered the story and we collectively cry out: "The world should not be like this! Children should not be abused, senior adults should not get Alzheimer's, missionaries should not be tortured!" Or on a more personal level we might protest: "Why me? What did I do to deserve this?"[6]

Thankfully, the fall is not the final theme in the story of God, for although we are fallen and now suffer, we are not forgotten by God. In loving grace, God keeps us as his image bearers. Sin and decay do not change our worth or value as human beings. One theologian described it this way:

> Yet we must remember that even fallen, sinful man has the status of being in God's image. . . . Every single human being, no matter how much the image of God is marred by sin, or illness, or weakness, or age, or any other disability, still has the status of being in God's image and therefore must be treated with the dignity and respect that is due to God's image-bearer. This has profound implications for our conduct toward others. It means that people of every race deserve equal dignity and rights. It means that elderly people, those seriously ill, . . . and unborn children

*deserve full protection and honor as human beings. If we ever deny our
unique status in creation as God's only image bearers, we will soon begin
to depreciate the value of human life, will tend to see humans as merely
a higher form of animal, and will begin to treat others as such. We will
also lose much of our sense of the meaning of life.*[7]

Alzheimer's strips away our worldly identity, but a person is valuable for who they are, not simply for what they can contribute. We are more than the sum of our memories. Even when we have nothing left to offer others, we still have value to God, and nothing can change that. The world looks at a person like Henry, whom we described at the start of this chapter, and sees him as irrelevant and unproductive. But the world does not see him as God sees him. Henry is a child of God, created in the image of God, who matters to God. God sent his own Son to suffer and die on his behalf, to make him a new creation. The biblical story tells us not just of creation and fall, but also how God restores our community with him and will one day bring an end to our suffering.

> Even when we have nothing left to offer others, we still have value to God, and nothing can change that.

Who Is God Making Us to Be?

As you can see, a biblical perspective on dementia is quite different from the typical way we think about this disease. Yes, Alzheimer's is bewildering, confusing, and painful, and it often leads to a cruel ending of this life. Putting our hope in God and his promises does not mean we will escape suffering. The Scriptures rightly note that we hope for "what we do not yet have," placing our hopes and our future dreams in what is unseen today. The stories of the Bible are filled with people who hope in God yet cry out to him in their suffering.

What changes is that our identity is no longer tied to what we can do or contribute; it is tied to who God is making us to be because of what Christ did. We are redeemed, bought from slavery to sin and death at the cost of Christ's own suffering. We are described as a new creation. Though the fall ruptured the relationship between God and his people, and brought with it great suffering, this relationship is restored through the suffering of Christ.

> So from now on we regard no one from a worldly point of view. Though we once regarded Christ in this way, we do so no longer. Therefore, if anyone is in Christ, the new creation has come: The old has gone, the new is here! All this is from God, who reconciled us to himself through Christ and gave us the ministry of reconciliation. (2 Corinthians 5:16–18)

The process of aging and the onset of dementia remind us that we live in a dual reality. While our bodies and brains fade, God has declared that we are a new creation with a new identity. Rooted in our identity in Christ, we are in the process of being transformed into someone new, a secure identity that will never fade away. The words of Scripture remind us that our identity is rooted in Christ; our true life is hidden in him (Colossians 3:3). In the words of Graeme Goldsworthy:

> *Christ, then, becomes our other identity, our alter ego. We possess and know this other self only by faith, hence we "live by faith, not by sight" (2 Cor. 5:7). Consequently, we have died with Christ and have been buried with him (Rom. 6:3–11; Gal. 2:19–20; Col. 2:12, 20). We have also been raised with him (Rom. 6:4–5, 11; 1 Cor. 15:22; Eph. 2:6) and we have ascended to the right hand of the Father with him (Eph. 2:6). In Christ we are a new creation (2 Cor. 5:17). None of these things are goals for us to achieve for they already exist perfectly in Christ on our behalf.*[8]

We have done nothing to achieve this identity and hope, nor can we do anything to earn it, which is good news for those who feel as if they can no longer help themselves. God accomplished all of this through Christ, and he promises that he "will carry it on to completion until the day of Christ Jesus" (Philippians 1:6) when we are fully restored.

> While our bodies and brains fade, God has declared that we are a new creation with a new identity.

When Alzheimer's manifests itself, we tend to forget these things. We forget that Henry is not primarily an "Alzheimer's patient"; he is a child of God, created in God's image. Although his body and brain have been dramatically affected by the fallen world, his identity in Christ is secure. Christ himself endured suffering on Henry's behalf that he might become a new creation, fully restored one day.

Where Is Our Hope in the Present?

God Fully Knows Us

Henry has an identity and value in Christ that can never be taken from him. But what hope does this offer him in the present? How does God meet Henry in the difficulties and suffering of dementia?[9]

One of the frustrating and frightening aspects of dementia is our inability to understand why people do the things they do. We often cannot understand why someone hides money in places and forgets about it. We don't understand why they wake up yelling in the middle of the night or drive off to an unknown location, hours from home.

Even though a person can become confused because of an impaired memory, that person still has real needs, feelings, and longings. This is key to understanding the behavioral challenges that occur in people with dementia. As people lose their ability to communicate with words, they have more difficulty expressing their needs, whether physical, emotional, or spiritual. The expression of these needs sometimes comes out in agitated behavior, wandering, crying, or aggression.[10] Caregivers can lovingly serve those with Alzheimer's by trying to understand the underlying need that is prompting the behavior.[11] Often, we only know and understand this partially. Yet even when we don't fully know what is in the heart and mind of the person with Alzheimer's, we can take comfort in knowing that there is One who fully knows us all.

J. I. Packer writes about the comfort we have in being known by God:

> What matters supremely, therefore, is not, in the last analysis, the fact that I know God, but the larger fact which underlies it — the fact that *he knows me*. I am graven on the palms of his hands [Isaiah 49:16]. I am never out of his mind. All my knowledge of

him depends on his sustained initiative in knowing me. I know him because he first knew me, and continues to know me. He knows me as a friend, one who loves me; and there is no moment when his eye is off me, or his attention distracted from me, and no moment, therefore, when his care falters.

This is momentous knowledge. There is unspeakable comfort—the sort of comfort that energizes, be it said, not enervates—in knowing that God is constantly taking knowledge of me in love and watching over me for my good. There is tremendous relief in knowing that his love to me is utterly realistic, based at every point on prior knowledge of the worst about me, so that no discovery now can disillusion him about me, in the way I am so often disillusioned about myself, and quench his determination to bless me.[12]

Caregivers often experience frustration—even anger—in trying to know and understand the mind and heart of the person with dementia that they care for. The truth is that there is much we will never know. But God knows. God knows the depths of our hearts and minds, even when they are chaotic and disordered. God knows our secret shame, the guilt of old sins, the pain of bitter disappointments, and the dizzying confusion of not knowing who we are, what day it is, or who is taking care of us. Whether you are dealing with dementia or with the physical and emotional demands of caregiving, you can rest in the fact that God knows and loves you fully as a unique individual. Nothing about you—what you've done or left undone, what you've remembered, or what you've forgotten—can change this.

> God knows and loves you fully as a unique individual. Nothing about you — what you've done or left undone, what you've remembered, or what you've forgotten — can change this.

In the Psalms, we are told that God knew us "in the womb," and he knit us together with care and love. If God knew us in this state, even before our own self-awareness, then he certainly knows us in the loss we experience in dementia. Take a moment to read and meditate on the comforting words of Psalm 139:

You have searched me, LORD,
*   and you know me.*
You know when I sit and when I rise;
*   you perceive my thoughts from afar.*
You discern my going out and my lying down;
*   you are familiar with all my ways.*
Before a word is on my tongue
*   you, LORD, know it completely. (vv. 1–4)*

When we consider our spirituality and faith walk we tend to be focused on what we do and say, and this can be a problem for people with progressive dementia. But this passage offers us very good news—God knows us, even before we act or speak.

You hem me in behind and before,
*   and you lay your hand upon me.*
Such knowledge is too wonderful for me,
*   too lofty for me to attain. (vv. 5–6)*

The knowledge that God has of us is difficult to understand, as the psalmist says. Not everything the Lord does or promises to us will be easy for us to comprehend, but that should not lead us to discount it. We can thankfully celebrate that God's ways are higher and better than ours when this world is confusing and painful.

Where can I go from your Spirit?
*   Where can I flee from your presence?*
If I go up to the heavens, you are there;
*   if I make my bed in the depths, you are there.*
If I rise on the wings of the dawn,
*   if I settle on the far side of the sea,*
even there your hand will guide me,
*   your right hand will hold me fast. (vv. 7–10)*

We cannot escape the presence of God. Wherever we go, the Lord will hold us fast, in the highest and lowest moments of our life.

If I say, "Surely the darkness will hide me
*   and the light become night around me,"*
even the darkness will not be dark to you;

the night will shine like the day,
  for darkness is as light to you. (vv. 11–12)

Even the seeming darkness of severe Alzheimer's disease does not separate us from the Lord and his love.

For you created my inmost being;
  you knit me together in my mother's womb.
I praise you because I am fearfully and wonderfully made;
  your works are wonderful,
  I know that full well.
My frame was not hidden from you
  when I was made in the secret place,
  when I was woven together in the depths of the earth.
Your eyes saw my unformed body;
  all the days ordained for me were written in your book
  before one of them came to be.
How precious to me are your thoughts, God!
  How vast is the sum of them!
Were I to count them,
  they would outnumber the grains of sand—
  when I awake, I am still with you. (vv. 13–18)

God is all knowing and he is all present. When Henry groans in the confusion of Alzheimer's, God is with him. Henry may not understand his groans, but God does, and he also understands the deepest longings of Henry's heart. And God doesn't stop with merely knowing and understanding Henry. He responds to him—in grace.

God Extends Grace in Our Groaning

God provides grace for those with Alzheimer's and other dementias. God's Word provides us with hope, even in our darkest hour, though we may not always see it. Sometimes what we see is not as important as what we do not see. Paul describes this:

I consider that our present sufferings are not worth comparing with the glory that will be revealed in us. For the creation waits in eager expectation for the children of God to be revealed. For the creation

was subjected to frustration, not by its own choice, but by the will
of the one who subjected it, in hope that the creation itself will be
liberated from its bondage to decay and brought into the freedom
and glory of the children of God. (Romans 8:18–21)

Those who have spent any time around people with advanced
dementia know of the "bondage to decay" Paul writes about here.
Conditions like Alzheimer's disease have such a hold on a person that
it can seem like a form of bondage—that the person is a slave to the
disease. Yet while there are great changes in their memory, personality, and behavior, there is still an underlying reality and an enduring
aspect of their identity that cannot be taken away. The footnote to
Romans 8:10 in the NIV tells us: "But if Christ is in *you, your body
is dead because of sin, yet your spirit is alive* because of righteousness"
(emphasis mine). Despite the effect of the curse upon our physical
bodies, these individuals remain children of God, created in his image,
and their identity and their life is still rooted securely in Christ. We
may be tempted to doubt this when a person becomes incontinent,
combative, agitated, and aggressive, but again listen to Paul:

> We know that the whole creation has been groaning as in the pains
> of childbirth right up to the present time. Not only so, but we our-
> selves, who have the firstfruits of the Spirit, groan inwardly as we
> wait eagerly for our adoption to sonship, the redemption of our bod-
> ies. For in this hope we were saved. But hope that is seen is no hope
> at all. Who hopes for what they already have? But if we hope for
> what we do not yet have, we wait for it patiently. (Romans 8:22–25)

People with dementia know this groaning. Seeking life through
the fog and confusion of dementia, they groan in frustration, both
inwardly (as the passage indicates) and outwardly. Deep within they
may recall a time when they were free from the weight of memory
impairment and confusion, and they may long for a better day. Caregivers will also groan as they long for behavioral challenges to stop, as
they long for a return to the way things were, and as they long for the
person to remember. Both the person with dementia and the caregiver
eagerly await the redemption and restoration of their bodies. As Paul

tells us, we wait for something we do not yet see and do not yet have, but this does not change the reality of our hope. Waiting and hoping requires faith, but thankfully we do not wait alone.

> In the same way, the Spirit helps us in our weakness. We do not know what we ought to pray for, but the Spirit himself intercedes for us through wordless groans. And he who searches our hearts knows the mind of the Spirit, because the Spirit intercedes for God's people in accordance with the will of God. (Romans 8:26–27)

The grace of God is evident in the way he responds to us in our weakness. Here Paul explains that we sometimes suffer so greatly that we don't even know what we ought to pray for. In these times, the Holy Spirit prays for us "through wordless groans." The Spirit intercedes for us when we cannot think of the words to pray. If you are caring for a person with dementia and find yourself overwhelmed, seemingly unable to do anything, this passage is for you.

It is also a word of hope to the person who has dementia. In their weakness, the Spirit intercedes with wordless groans on their behalf as well. Sometimes, a person advances to a stage when articulating needs and prayers becomes difficult, if not impossible. But here we are told that the Lord continues to search and know their hearts, interceding on their behalf with these wordless groans in accordance with God's will. Our faith is in a God who is good, loving, and compassionate. Even when we are unable to speak — perhaps because we are overwhelmed and weak or the disease has severely damaged our brain — we are promised that God still searches our hearts, seeing our innermost thoughts, fears, and hopes, and he responds with prayers on our behalf. God's grace is so amazing. He gives us what we need when we are too weak or confused to ask for it ourselves. In Alzheimer's disease we are reminded that God knows us better than we know ourselves.

Some worry that a Christian who develops Alzheimer's disease will forget the Lord and somehow lose their salvation. One pastor who has worked with families caring for loved ones with dementia noted that problem behaviors would sometimes lead families and friends to question the faith of the person with dementia. They would note the changes in behavior and would be tempted to think that these behaviors were the real indicators of the person's faith, rather than the life of faith they had lived to that point. But we need to remember that both our salvation and ongoing faith are the result of the work of God, rather than our own faithfulness. When the ability of a loved one to think and act is damaged, we must cling to this good news, that God has called them and they belong to him.

We should also try to have humility in judging the heart of someone who has descended into the depths of dementia, leaving it to God to search their heart. Even in those who are not suffering from dementia, there are times when we forget and the Holy Spirit must help us to remember the truth. The Scriptures tell us that the Spirit intercedes for us as well, and there is no reason to believe this is any different for people with dementia. God is committed to continuing the work he began, and calling to himself those who are his:

> And we know that in all things God works for the good of those who love him, who have been called according to his purpose. For those God foreknew he also predestined to be conformed to the image of his Son, that he might be the firstborn among many brothers and sisters. And those he predestined, he also called; those he called, he also justified; those he justified, he also glorified. (Romans 8:28–30)

Dementia Cannot Separate Us

Ultimately, we have the promise that nothing can separate us from the great love of God in Christ. Paul says this in Romans 8:35–39:

> Who shall separate us from the love of Christ? Shall trouble or hardship or persecution or famine or nakedness or danger or sword? As it is written:
>
> > *"For your sake we face death all day long;*
> > *we are considered as sheep to be slaughtered."*
>
> No, in all these things we are more than conquerors through him who loved us. For I am convinced that neither death nor life, neither angels nor demons, neither the present nor the future, nor any powers, neither height nor depth, nor anything else in all

creation, will be able to separate us from the love of God that is in Christ Jesus our Lord.

Though Alzheimer's disease is a frightening and powerful enemy, the promise of God is greater: nothing can separate those who are in Christ from the love and grace of God. Not the plaques and tangles of Alzheimer's disease, not the memory impairment observed on psychological testing, not the behavioral problems, the aggression, confusion, or even the apparent forgetting of the Lord can separate us from him.

You may worry deeply about the faith of your loved one, but take deep comfort in knowing that when they turn toward the Lord, he runs toward them. We see this in the response of the father in the parable of the prodigal son. "But while he [the son] was still a long way off, his father saw him and was filled with compassion for him; he ran to his son, threw his arms around him and kissed him" (Luke 15:20). All of this happens before the son can even speak. It's as if the father knows his son's heart and is ready to take him back.

Those with dementia need not speak. Not even the disease's ravages can separate us from God's radical grace and love. We don't really know what turning to him looks like in deep dementia, but we can know that God doesn't require that we have the right words. He looks at what is within, at the heart. We may never know how the person hears him, whether as a still, small voice or gentle whisper deep within (1 Kings 19:12) or as a bright blinding light (Acts 9:3). Some mysteries will never be solved before we reach heaven and meet him face-to-face (1 Corinthians 13:12). But while we wait, God asks us to remember his promises and his presence, so that we can experience his peace that surpasses all understanding.

One caregiver shared this account with me recently:

During my last visit, I was seeking God with questions: "Can she [mother] access you? Can she access her long-held faith? Can she receive comfort from you, Lord?" Her social skills have deteriorated such that we don't have much of a two-sided conversation. "Can she converse with you and share her fears, needs—things she can't share with me anymore?" God graciously reminded me that relating to him is not dependent on her ability to access him. His ability to connect with her is unchanged. Do I not believe that the creator and sustainer of the universe is creative enough to be able to cut through her fog and relate to her personally? As she napped (something she does a lot of these days) I prayed that God's presence would fill her living space. And then I asked him, "What about her last moments? What if she is afraid …?"

In that moment, God answered me: "I'll be here with her, and she will know it. Have no fear."

Because grace is extended and received as a gift, we can be confident that the Lord holds on to his children. "The Lord knows those who are his" (2 Timothy 2:19). As a caregiver, when you feel that the person you love may be lost, listen to how Jesus talked about his children and followers in this parable:

> Then Jesus told them this parable: "Suppose one of you has a hundred sheep and loses one of them. Doesn't he leave the ninety-nine in the open country and go after the lost sheep until he finds it? And when he finds it, he joyfully puts it on his shoulders and goes home. Then he calls his friends and neighbors together and says, 'Rejoice with me; I have found my lost sheep.' I tell you that in the same way there will be more rejoicing in heaven over one sinner who repents than over ninety-nine righteous persons who do not need to repent." (Luke 15:3–7)

Jesus reminds us that the Lord cares about each person, just as a shepherd cares for each of his sheep. When one is lost, he searches until he finds it. Here, as always, it is God who initiates the search. He seeks us. When you fear that your loved one is no longer seeking God, remember that it is God who first sought us, even before we first believed.

God Promises Restoration

Although death seems like the end, it is really just the beginning of a longer and sweeter reality that will last forever. This life is filled with great trouble and, by God's grace, some joy. But the joy and trouble of this life are nothing compared to the eternal joy we will know when

God makes all things new, gives us our new bodies, and we experience his rest.

Though the troubles of Alzheimer's seem unending, the struggle is for just a short time. God promises us that our current sufferings are as nothing compared to the joys we will experience if we put our trust in him.

> Therefore we do not lose heart. Though outwardly we are wasting away, yet inwardly we are being renewed day by day. For our light and momentary troubles are achieving for us an eternal glory that far outweighs them all. So we fix our eyes not on what is seen, but on what is unseen, since what is seen is temporary, but what is unseen is eternal. (2 Corinthians 4:16–18)

One caregiver shared that she coped with the challenges she faced by continually reminding herself that everything she was dealing with was temporary, no matter how hard it got.

God's grace supplies redemption and a hope for restoration in the future. We are promised a new life in which we will live without frustration, decay, and death and in which we can truly glorify God and live in the beauty of love for him and those around us. When you consider a loved one whose mind and very being seem ravaged by Alzheimer's disease, take hope not just that they have an inheritance awaiting them in heaven, but that the God who created and redeemed them will also restore them to such a state that he will rejoice over them. Even though they will experience trials for the duration of this life, God will be with them guiding them into the beautiful hope awaiting them in the next.

• •

FOR FURTHER REFLECTION

In this chapter we learned how God fully knows and reaches us even when we can't speak and others can't seem to understand us. When we can't speak a word of prayer, he prays on our behalf. When we groan under the weight of sorrow and suffering, the Holy Spirit groans with us and intercedes on our behalf. When we seek the Lord, it is because the Holy Spirit moved and prompted first.

- If you care for someone with Alzheimer's, how does this change the way you see their spiritual life? How might this influence the way you see them and provide care?

- How does this knowledge of God's provision influence your own faith?

• •

Chapter 5

THE CHALLENGES OF GIVING CARE

ONE OF THE CHALLENGES FOR FAMILIES affected by Alzheimer's disease is recognizing what is happening and knowing when to step in. As people experience memory changes they will lose some capacity to take care of themselves. This can be difficult for those who love them, not only because more care is needed, but because it is surprisingly hard to see what is happening in the early stages of the disease.

Even those who are familiar with dementia and know how to help others often find it challenging when it hits them personally. Although Karen was involved in ministry to people with memory failure and their caregivers, she shared with me that she failed to recognize the symptoms in her own mother as they slowly developed over a five-year period. Karen told me she was in denial, unwilling to acknowledge what was happening. Karen initially attributed the subtle changes to grief because her mother had lost her husband a few years earlier. It wasn't until her mother showed more noticeable symptoms that she was able to see what was happening. One Christmas, for example, Karen received a bank gift card from her mother, instead of the typical cash gift that she had always given in the past. When the family tried to use the cards they discovered that there was no money on them. Though it could have been an innocent mistake, it seemed unusual. She began to reflect on the past few years and realized that other, equally subtle changes had been taking place. Her mother hadn't been managing her money as well as she had in the past. She had some rental property and increasingly needed help with it. All of these added together raised some alarms with Karen. She took her mother to the doctor who diagnosed her with vascular dementia, a form of dementia caused by strokes or other blockages or ruptures within the blood vessels in the brain.

After the diagnosis, the changes were easier to see. Karen saw a noticeable decline in her mother's ability to remember things. Soon the person who cared for the caregivers found herself serving as a primary caregiver. Karen found herself doing more and more for her mother until she felt like she was doing everything—laundry, meals, medication management. She would even get her mother up and dressed for the day before heading to work. Like many caregivers, she found herself in the dual role of caring for her mother and working a full-time job outside the home. Her physical and emotional resources were becoming depleted.

Being a caregiver takes a toll, but the needs of caregivers are often hidden behind the more obvious needs of the person suffering the disease. In fact, for decades, the needs of caregivers were neglected. They became the hidden victims of dementia. While dementia treatments focused on trying to reduce the symptoms of dementia, healthcare providers failed to recognize the physical and relational burdens carried by the families providing the care. Over the past two decades, research has confirmed just how difficult things can be for a caregiver.

Today, everyone you talk with is *busy*. Whenever I ask people how they are doing, they tell me they're busy.[1] We live in a mobile society, constantly on the go, often without a spare moment's peace. Is it any surprise that we are unable to consistently remember the *why* behind the frantic activities of our lives? What is life about? Who and what are we living for? In our busy, hurried lives, we forget to spend time in the presence of God. Even when we pause to remember, we do so in such a cursory fashion that it fails to penetrate the heart. We may remember God as a concept, but we fail to remember the goodness we've experienced in meeting with him as a loving, powerful, and caring person. In our stress-induced forgetting, we forfeit the peace God offers us.

As busy as our lives can be today, consider what it would be like to add to all of this the full-time care of a person who is declining mentally and physically. You may already know what this is like. They forget to take their medication, pay the bills, change their clothes or shower, sometimes even to eat. They get their days and nights confused, napping on and off during the day and walking around the house all night. They are prone to wander off, leaving you unable to sleep at night for fear that they will leave the house, heading into the cold of the night and unable to find their way back to the warmth of the house.[2] At some point, they may need help eating or putting on their clothes. Take the busyness of life and then add this to your plate—it's a recipe for burnout.

Perhaps, though, your busy and hectic days are behind you. You've worked hard for decades and anticipated a peaceful rest in retirement. You persevered through long hours and sacrificed much in hopes of seeing the world or buying a vacation home in a warmer place, or even just enjoying an extended time of rest. You scrimped and saved in hope for something better. Now, as you approach retirement, your spouse seems to be changing. She repeats herself often, and perhaps even more concerning, she doesn't want to leave the house, has stopped contacting her friends, and seems confused. Nonetheless, you decide to take the first trip you had planned together. Things seem fine until the second night. She wakes up confused about where she is, and after you explain, she still has a terrified look in her eyes. You begin to see your dreams disappearing, and as the days push on, you feel a sense of dread as you start to believe that your beloved spouse is slipping away. You feel helpless, like there is nothing you can do.

These scenarios describe life for nearly 15 million people across America who provide an estimated 17.4 billion hours of care each year.

If they were paid for this work it would cost 210 billion dollars. Statistics provided by Michael Castleman and his colleagues integrated the results from three separate caregiver studies and reported that 55 percent of caregivers are spouses and 35 percent are adult children (most of whom are daughters or daughters-in-law). The remaining 10 percent of caregivers are siblings, close friends, or paid caregivers. Seventy-five percent of all caregivers are women. One-third of these caregivers are the only person providing care for the person with dementia — that is, a third of the 15 million caregivers are doing it alone.[3]

Giving Care to Others

On average, caregivers spend seventy hours a week providing care. This number is as high as a hundred hours per week among those who do not hold a job and averages about forty hours per week among those who do hold a job. In reality, caregiving represents a second full-time job. Those who hold a job while caregiving report that the demands often interfere with their work. They often find they need to take days off from work, which can directly affect their career advancement. The additional time spent giving care is compounded by the nature of the tasks involved. Seventy percent of caregivers say they feel unable to leave their loved one alone, even in their home. Up to two-thirds report that the person they care for needs help with such basic functions as getting dressed, using the bathroom, and bathing.[4]

Caregiving typically occurs in the context of a long-standing family relationship, either between a husband and wife or between a parent and child. As a result, each caregiving relationship is unique. Still, there are some common themes and challenges in every caregiving relationship. Understanding these will help us learn how to give better care to those suffering from dementia, and how to care for the caregivers themselves.

Types of Help Provided by Caregivers

Whether the person you care for needs little or extensive care depends on their ability to complete their activities of daily living. Professional

Instrumental Activities of Daily Living (IADLs)	Basic Activities of Daily Living (ADLs)
Managing money	Bathing
Taking medicine appropriately	Hygiene
Grocery shopping	Eating
Driving	Getting dressed
Using telephone and other technology	Walking and moving around
Housework	Getting in and out of bed

care providers refer to this in terms of basic "activities of daily living" (ADLs) and "instrumental activities of daily living" (IADLs). Examples of these activities are listed in the table.

If your loved one has dementia you are likely providing help with at least one of the IADLs, and as they move into more advanced stages you will find yourself providing greater assistance with basic ADLs as well.

When we consider the changes in brain function and memory, it is not hard to see why individuals have trouble with these activities of daily living. Memory problems lead people to forget to take their medication or take it too many times in one day. They forget to pay their bills. Slower thinking and diminished attention can lead to unsafe driving. As a result, family members must step in to provide supervision and assistance with these tasks to ensure the safety and well-being of their loved one.

Providing this kind of care requires time. Caregivers find their schedules slowly filling up with responsibilities as they provide for more and more of the tasks of daily living. This places great strain on them. It is tiring and difficult because there are only so many hours in each day, and these responsibilities are being added to an already full schedule. Not surprisingly, studies of caregivers show that they experience considerable weariness and exhaustion.[5]

Behavioral Problems

As stressful as it is to help with the tasks of daily living, another set of challenges can lead to even more distress and greater feelings of burden and grief. Most individuals with dementia also experience changes in their behavior and personality. They may begin to wander off, show aggressive behaviors like hitting or yelling, appear restless, or display agitation. They may begin following loved ones around the home and cannot be left alone. Some also experience mood changes like depression and anxiety. Others experience hallucinations (seeing or hearing things that others don't) and delusions (false beliefs that don't change despite evidence to the contrary). Some also become less inhibited and may say or do things that they never or rarely would have in the past. This includes cursing, insults, and sexually inappropriate behaviors. Still others experience apathy—they don't seem to care about anything or anyone anymore, and it is difficult to get them to do anything, including getting out of bed or taking a shower. Up to 90 percent of people with dementia will experience at least one of these problems at some time in the progression of their disease.[6]

These behaviors increase the burdens placed on the caregiver, leading to a reduced quality of life.[7] Research on caregiving has consistently shown that these aspects of dementia care are the most upsetting for people and can lead caregivers to experience grief, even though the person is still living.[8] Caregivers may grieve the loss of the way the person was, and many report that it seems as if they are living with or caring for a different person. Others grieve because the life they once had is now gone and they recognize that the end of the person's life is approaching faster than they had thought.

The Impact on Caregivers

Some caregivers find themselves facing tough choices as the demands and responsibilities increase. Some must make sacrifices, choosing between the time and energy needed to care for a parent and the other commitments in their life—even raising their own children.[9] Some families choose to devote greater time and resources toward their children, while others devote more toward their parents, but in either case they feel torn between the two.[10] This can prompt role reversals in which the adult now ends up taking care of his or her parents.

At some point, most caregivers admit that they feel absolutely alone, as if no one understands what they are going through.

> At some point, most caregivers admit that they feel absolutely alone, as if no one understands what they are going through.

They feel that the weight and responsibility for this person rests completely on them. When one woman described the challenges of caring for her mother, who was in the moderate stages of dementia, to her support group, they offered suggestion after suggestion, all of them born out of their own years of caregiving experience. Yet for each suggestion, the woman calmly but sadly replied that she had tried it and it hadn't helped. She was discouraged and depressed. Many caregivers live in quiet desperation like this, feeling as though they are alone and helpless. Even in a room of sympathetic caregivers, this woman felt alone. All of the things that had worked for others seemed to fail in her situation. It felt hopeless.

In the midst of their loneliness, discouragement, depression, grief, and fatigue, many caregivers cry out to the Lord for mercy. And many find that in doing this they encounter the grace and provision of God. The words of this prayer are particularly fitting for caregivers in need of help:

I am weary, Lord ... bone tired.
Weary to the point of tears, and past them.
Your Word says you never grow weary;
But I know you understand weariness
Because once you dragged a heavy cross
up a long lonely hill.
Many times you had nowhere to lay your head—
And people who needed you pressed upon you
by day and by night.
My reservoir is depleted, almost dry.

For longer than I can remember I've been
  dredging from its sludgy underside
Giving myself and my loved ones the leftovers
  of a life occupied with endless tasks.
The elastic of my life is so stretched out of shape
  that it doesn't snap back anymore.
Just once I'd like to say "It is finished," like you did.
But you said it just before you died.
I guess my job won't be over till my life is
  and that's okay Lord,
    if you'll just give me strength to live it.
Deliver me from this limbo of half-life;
  Not just surviving, but thriving.
You who know all, you who know me
  far better than I know myself—
Deposit to my account that as I spend myself
  there may be always more to draw from.
Give me strength
  To rest without guilt . . .
    To run without frenzy . . .
      To soar like an eagle
Over the broad breathless canyons of the life
you still have for me both here and beyond.[11]

Crying Out in the Night

Nighttime brings special challenges to caregivers. They may need to watch a person wandering around the house. For others, nighttime is filled with silence, leaving the caregiver with his thoughts about the care he provided that day or fears about what will be needed tomorrow. These anxieties, along with the guilt and hopeless feelings, can be particularly strong in the darkness of night. Psalm 77 captures this aspect of the caregiving experience quite well:

I cried out to God for help;
  I cried out to God to hear me.
When I was in distress, I sought the LORD;

at night I stretched out untiring hands,
and I would not be comforted.
I remembered you, God, and I groaned;
I meditated, and my spirit grew faint.
You kept my eyes from closing;
I was too troubled to speak.
I thought about the former days,
the years of long ago;
I remembered my songs in the night.
My heart meditated and my spirit asked:
"Will the LORD *reject forever?*
Will he never show his favor again?
Has his unfailing love vanished forever?
Has his promise failed for all time?
Has God forgotten to be merciful?
Has he in anger withheld his compassion?" (vv. 1–9)

Here the psalmist is awake, unable to sleep, and clearly suffering. He feels so alone that he thinks God may have forgotten him. Nights can be like that. He remembers better days and compares them to his current lot. He wonders if God's love and compassion have run out and questions whether God will keep his promises.

But in the midst of these questions and doubts, the remembrance of God and his faithfulness turns his experience from loneliness to comfort:

Then I thought, "To this I will appeal:
the years when the Most High stretched out his right hand.
I will remember the deeds of the LORD;
yes, I will remember your miracles of long ago.
I will consider all your works
and meditate on all your mighty deeds."
Your ways, God, are holy.
What god is as great as our God?
You are the God who performs miracles;
you display your power among the peoples.
With your mighty arm you redeemed your people,
the descendants of Jacob and Joseph.
The waters saw you, God,

the waters saw you and writhed;
the very depths were convulsed.
The clouds poured down water,
the heavens resounded with thunder;
your arrows flashed back and forth.
Your thunder was heard in the whirlwind,
your lightning lit up the world;
the earth trembled and quaked.
Your path led through the sea,
your way through the mighty waters,
though your footprints were not seen.
You led your people like a flock
by the hand of Moses and Aaron. (vv. 10–20)

God does not sleep. When you are awake in the night, filled with fear and worry or watching over a parent or spouse with dementia, remember that God is not sleeping either. He is with you. He is watching over you. (Psalm 121)

The Groans of Giving Care

God wants caregivers to remember that he is present, even in these dark places, and he lovingly encourages them to bring their "groans" to him. Groaning is a common way of expressing the emotions behind suffering in both the Old and New Testaments. We are told that the people of Israel groaned under the oppression of the Egyptians (Exodus 6:5). Groaning is also a response to sorrow, fatigue, lack of rest, and physical affliction (see Psalms 6:6, 31:10, 32:3; Jeremiah 45:3). In the book of Romans, groaning is used to describe the longing that the creation has for renewal, a groaning similar to the groans of a woman in the pains of childbirth (Romans 8:22). As we saw earlier, the Holy Spirit also groans in prayer on our behalf (Romans 8:26).

Know that there may come a time when you feel so burdened and overwhelmed that you don't know what to pray. Words may fail you. Take comfort knowing that God has anticipated this. The groans of

God's people express their deep longing for the Lord and for his restoration, his salvation. Part of our groaning is in anticipation of this future hope, a better reality where pain and suffering will be no more (2 Corinthians 5). We hope for this with anticipation, waiting in faith, not by sight (v. 7). We live in the tension between the victory of what God has already done for us in Christ, yet knowing that some promises remain to be fulfilled.

> There may come a time when you feel so burdened and overwhelmed that you don't know what to pray.

As they care for their loved ones, many people speak of finding God's grace in unexpected places, like a cup of cool water in the midst of a dry desert wilderness. Like water pouring out a rock, they are reminded of the goodness of God, his grace in the midst of trial. You may not see this grace in your life right now, but if you watch and listen for it, you will find it. It often comes in surprising ways. Most caregivers report seeing God's grace in the small but meaningful aspects of their caring relationships. They hear God speaking his love and comfort to them in

> ... the words of a husband whispering his appreciation to his "loving bride."
> ... a new friendship for a parent who is living in a nursing home.
> ... singing an old hymn with Mom.
> ... watching God provide for new care needs in a long-distance caregiving relationship.
> ... knowing "the promise that God will be present through the rest of this journey in ways we cannot."
> ... hearing a spouse say, "I don't know what I would do without you."
> ... shared laughter and an enduring sense of humor.
> ... an hour or two of respite from ongoing caregiving.
> ... a poem, prayer, or devotion sent from a caring friend.
> ... a phone call from someone, just to check up.
> ... watching the sunrise.

... growing closer to a mother in her final years of dementia, and finally hearing her say, "I love you."

... learning to enjoy the moments and joy, and the small things in life that mean so much, like a smile.

You may groan for a new reality, but take heart as the psalmist does by remembering God's faithfulness in the past, even if you don't feel it right now. Remember what God has done in your life. Be specific. What experiences has he walked through with you? How have you experienced his goodness and provision? Remember what Christ has done for you and how this is linked to your promised future. Though the nights can be long, your loving God promises that his grace is new every morning. And though the waters of caregiving seem to rise endlessly, the Lord will be your hiding place. He will surround you with songs of deliverance:

> *Therefore let all the faithful pray to you*
> *while you may be found;*
> *surely the rising of the mighty waters*
> *will not reach them.*
> *You are my hiding place;*
> *you will protect me from trouble*
> *and surround me with songs of deliverance. (Psalm 32:6–7)*

Groaning vs. Grumbling

We have discussed the reality of groaning in the caregiving experience, the longings we have for restoration and for the Lord to work and intervene. But there is a critical difference here we need to note. Groaning is not grumbling. When we groan, we must learn to do it *without* grumbling, trusting in the faithfulness of God and his promises.

Groaning and grumbling can seem similar, but biblically they are quite different. Both are responses to suffering, but their sources and their direction are different. Groaning is a response to the weight of suffering, and it is directed toward God as an honest expression of pain, grief, and sorrow. Grumbling also reflects the weight of suffering, but it springs from anger and resentment toward God. It lacks a memory of his past faithfulness. Groaning expresses an element of hope in God, despite current sufferings, but grumbling reflects a lack of hope and faith and is accompanied by a sense of doom. In the Bible, we see that God responds to groaning with mercy, but he responds to grumbling with anger

> We can be confident that God hears and remembers us. He knows the cries of our hearts before we speak and calls us to lean on and trust in him.

and discipline. Still, even when we grumble there is hope. God is slow to anger, he does not forget his promises, and even in his discipline his goal is to draw his people to him in grace and pardon.

In the story of the Israelites wandering in the wilderness, we frequently encounter times when they grumbled to God. They often complained and did not believe that God's protection and provision for them was adequate (Exodus 16; Deuteronomy 1). Although God took them through challenging experiences to teach them to depend and rely upon him, they were quick to turn on him when the heat rose, rather than trusting that he would deliver them again. Grumbling is clearly something we should avoid, and we find this in the New Testament as well. In Philippians 2:14 and 1 Peter 4:9 we are explicitly reminded of this, encouraged to do everything, including offering hospitality to others, without complaining or grumbling.

You can experience the burden of caring for your loved one in many different ways. You may feel worn out and just plain tired at times. You may find yourself longing for the restoration of the one you love. Some grow bitter through the long hours of thankless care for someone who only responds with anger and paranoia. Grumbling is a sign that bitterness has developed in the heart. If you find you've been grumbling, confess it to the Lord and receive his mercy. Psalm 32 is a wonderful confession of sin for one who has felt the weight of suffering:

> *Blessed is the one*
> *whose transgressions are forgiven,*
> *whose sins are covered.*

Blessed is the one
  whose sin the LORD does not count against them
  and in whose spirit is no deceit.
When I kept silent,
  my bones wasted away
  through my groaning all day long.
For day and night
  your hand was heavy on me;
my strength was sapped
  as in the heat of summer.
Then I acknowledged my sin to you
  and did not cover up my iniquity.
I said, "I will confess
  my transgressions to the LORD."
And you forgave
  the guilt of my sin. (vv. 1–5)

Whether we groan or grumble, we can be confident that God hears and remembers us. He knows the cries of our hearts before we speak and calls us to lean on and trust in him.

FOR FURTHER REFLECTION

In this chapter we learned about the challenges of giving care.

- If you are a caregiver, what are the most difficult aspects in your experience? Where do you find yourself groaning for God's mercy and help? Where have you unexpectedly experienced his grace in the midst of this trial? Ask God to help you see and experience his grace today.

- If you aren't a caregiver, considering what you've read about caregiving, what do you think would be the most challenging for you personally? Ask God to show you how you might be able to serve a caregiver you know.

Chapter 6

GOD'S GRACE FOR CAREGIVERS

Having a parent with Alzheimer's is difficult. Having two parents with Alzheimer's is even worse. Trying to take care of them when they live five hundred miles away seems impossible. Yet this is the situation in which Samantha found herself. Her father had developed Alzheimer's ten years ago, and her mother had been caring for him as best she could. Samantha would visit them each month to cook, take care of bills and financial matters, coordinate any new care needs, and assess how they were doing. Eventually her father progressed to the point that her mother's aging body and mind were unable to keep up with his needs. He was placed in a memory-care unit.

Samantha's mother's caregiving over the last few years had taken a toll on her, and she was no longer doing well. Samantha hoped that her mother, who was also her best friend and closest confidant, might eventually begin to feel better. But she did not improve and had to be moved into an assisted-living facility. Not long after this, Samantha's father died.

Samantha traveled home more often to take care of her mother. She visited, made phone calls to make sure meals were delivered, and even hired personal care workers to help out. But it was never enough. Her mother grew increasingly forgetful. Eventually, she was diagnosed with Alzheimer's and moved into the same memory-care unit where her husband had died.

When the diagnosis came, Samantha felt the heavy emotional toll of caring for her mother. Even though her mother is still alive, she has begun grieving the loss of her relationship as a friend. At first, she says she "struggled to 'save her' from the obvious signs of the disease." Her initial caregiving efforts were a "feeble attempt at fixing and rescuing her."

When someone you love has dementia, the present seems large and out of control. The immediate problems dominate our hearts and minds, and we can forget that there is more to life. In this chapter, we will look at how it is possible to live and find strength in the present in light of what God has done for us in the past and what he has promised for our future. How does our present situation and our perspective change when we remember these things? How can we learn and grow in grace during this period?

I met with a pastor who lamented that he hasn't had much time to reflect on his experience of taking care of his father who has Alzheimer's. This pastor spends much of his time caring for both his father and for his mother, who is the primary caregiver. He does all this in addition to caring for his church and his own wife and children. He feels he has too much on his plate, with no time or energy left to even ask what God is teaching him and how he might use this time to form and shape him. Caregiving is like that. It takes everything you have and leaves you feeling drained of any energy or creativity or spiritual life.

Some caregivers cry out for God to remove their burden and take away the pain of caregiving. The apostle Paul also cried out to the Lord asking him to remove a burden from him in 2 Corinthians 12, and even though he called out many times, he didn't receive the reply he had hoped for. Instead, he discovered that God's grace can be found even in suffering. The Lord said to Paul, "My grace is sufficient for you, for my power is made perfect in weakness" (2 Corinthians 12:9). When we feel the weight of our earthly burdens, God calls us to trust him so that we can know his power and grace more deeply. Paul writes, "Therefore I will boast all the more gladly about my weaknesses, so that Christ's power may rest on me. That is why, for Christ's sake, I delight in weaknesses, in insults, in hardships, in persecutions, in difficulties. For when I am weak, then I am strong" (vv. 9–10).

As you sacrifice your strength on behalf of others, you can begin to experience the grace of Christ in this way as well. In our weakness, God tells us that we will find his strength for the tasks of everyday living. We can give glory to God in everyday, mundane tasks. We do this by relying on what God provides for us—his past provision, his present provision, and his future promises in Christ.

Christ, Our Caregiver

What has God provided for us? The gospel tells us that Christ humbled himself, living a sacrificial life crowned by the ultimate sacrifice of suffering and dying for us on the cross. Christ gave himself up to give us hope and a future (Jeremiah 29:11). The sacrifice of Christ secures excellent promises for our future and gives us a model for how to live in the present.

The New Testament is filled with passages that promise us a new hope in redemption through the forgiveness of sins and hope for full restoration in the future. Because of Christ's sacrifice, we have a hope that cannot fade or be taken from us. Here is the promise that Jesus shares with his followers:

> Do not let your hearts be troubled. You believe in God; believe also in me. My Father's house has many rooms; if that were not so, would I have told you that I am going there to prepare a place for you? And if I go and prepare a place for you, I will come back and take you to be with me that you also may be where I am. You know the way to the place where I am going. (John 14:1–4)

Jesus tells us that he is going away to prepare a new home for us and that we will go there to be with him one day. This is the promise of a new home, a new reality of life with God. Now I realize that this promise can seem disconnected from the daily reality of caregiving.

But in those moments when we feel like calling it quits, God calls us to press on, to keep our eyes fixed on what we have not yet attained. God *assures* us that this will be our reality and we can count on his word, even if it seems far off.

> But our citizenship is in heaven. And we eagerly await a Savior from there, the Lord Jesus Christ, who, by the power that enables him to bring everything under his control, will transform our lowly bodies so that they will be like his glorious body. (Philippians 3:20–21)

The Lord promises to restore our bodies and brains, transforming them to a glorious state. The ravaged brain of the person with Alzheimer's *will* be made new. The bodies of caregivers, filled with fatigue and weariness, *will* be made new. Today we long for this rest, like the Israelites longed for the Promised Land. And like the Israelites, we need to learn to trust the Lord's provision and his plan to take us home. We may wander in the wilderness for years, but we know with assurance that the Promised Land is our destination.

> As a caregiver, you can take comfort in the knowledge that you too have a caregiver, one who can surpassingly meet all of your needs. Christ is our caregiver.

Christ also promises us that we will not have to wait alone. Jesus promised to send his Holy Spirit to be among us, to comfort us, and to help us remember all that he has taught us. On those long nights and chaotic days, remember that God is with you through his Holy Spirit to guide you.

As a caregiver, you can take comfort in the knowledge that you too have a caregiver, one who can surpassingly meet all of your needs. Christ is our caregiver.

- He lived a sacrificial life, giving himself up for us.
- He humbled himself to serve us.
- He pursues us in grace, even when we resist his care. In our confusion, we may push him away when all he is trying to do is take care of us.
- He does not leave us alone and provides a helper for our needs.

Christ, Our Model

Ephesians 5 is a passage that teaches us how to incorporate what Christ has done for us into our present lives, including our caregiving: "Follow God's example, therefore, as dearly loved children and walk in the way of love, just as Christ loved us and gave himself up for us as a fragrant offering and sacrifice to God" (vv. 1–2).

God calls us to walk in the way of love. How? By remembering what Christ has done for us and following his example in the way we treat others. You make many sacrifices to provide care for someone with dementia. In a concrete way you are putting the needs of someone else before yourself. This is a practical and present expression of Christ's own sacrificial love, and we are called to live this way in imitation of Christ. Ephesians 5 tells us that we should give ourselves up for others as Christ did for his church. When we give of ourselves and give up parts of ourselves to provide for someone else who cannot provide for their own needs, we are proclaiming the gospel through our example.

One woman shared with me how she experienced this while caring for her husband with Alzheimer's disease:

> When we entered the world of Alzheimer's we already knew that life holds trials for the Christian. We had already experienced many of them ... so that was not a surprise. But it didn't prevent me from crying myself to sleep a lot of nights, or wondering how an extremely intelligent man whose life was always one of searching for new insights and information could have his eyes and his mind taken from him. It didn't prevent me from feeling as if I was sacrificing who I was in order to care for the man I love. I'm not talking a martyr complex, but with everything I had to give up, I sensed I was laying one more thing on the altar of love. Yet, I sensed—and knew—that the grace from my Lord was sufficient to carry me through. It didn't keep me from feeling lonely at times.

A caregiver must give up some of herself to serve another. You might be needed to help a person bathe, use the bathroom, or do other tasks that are unpleasant. This can take so much of your time that you have to give up other parts of your life, likely things that you enjoy or that are important to you. It is common for people to think,

"Why should I have to give this up for my family member?" In times like this, we need to recall the gospel and be grateful that Jesus did not respond this way to our sin. Instead of looking out for himself, Jesus put our needs first, giving himself to help us in our sin.

In addition to his once-for-all sacrificial death, Jesus modeled what it meant to be a servant. The greatest man who ever lived washed his disciples' feet, a task that was unpleasant and was viewed as something lowly, a task no one else wanted to do:

> "Do you understand what I have done for you?" he asked them. "You call me 'Teacher' and 'Lord,' and rightly so, for that is what I am. Now that I, your Lord and Teacher, have washed your feet, you also should wash one another's feet. I have set you an example that you should do as I have done for you. Very truly I tell you, no servant is greater than his master, nor is a messenger greater than the one who sent him. Now that you know these things, you will be blessed if you do them." (John 13:12–17)

Not only did Jesus embrace the lowest of tasks to serve others, he encouraged his disciples to follow his example. He promises us that we will be blessed when we do. I realize that something inside of us chafes at the idea of being a servant, especially when we are unlikely to receive any thanks from the ones we serve. We live in a culture that glorifies the great, the strong, and the beautiful. It's rare to hear anyone praise the husband who gives up his work or freedom to stay at home to care for his wife,[1] or the daughter who patiently answers the anxious questions of her father over and over again as they slowly walk around the block.

> Not so with you. Instead, whoever wants to become great among you must be your servant, and whoever wants to be first must be your slave—just as the Son of Man did not come to be served, but to serve, and to give his life as a ransom for many. (Matthew 20:26–28; see also Mark 10:43–44)

The way of Christ—the way of love—turns our natural selfish tendencies upside down. Jesus tells us that the pursuit of greatness is not found in pleasing ourselves but in being a humble servant of others. Jesus taught that those who seek to exalt themselves will one day be humbled, while those who humble themselves in service today will be exalted one day (Matthew 23:12). Philippians 2 also encourages us to imitate Christ in his humility and servant nature:

> In humility value others above yourselves, not looking to your own interests but each of you to the interests of the others. *In your relationships with one another, have the same mindset as Christ Jesus*: Who, being in very nature God, did not consider equality with God something to be used to his own advantage; rather, he made himself nothing by taking the very nature of a servant." (vv. 3–7; italics added)

If you find yourself feeling burdened, worn out, discouraged, or even humiliated by the tasks you've taken on as a caregiver, remember the example of Christ. He was the lowliest of servants when he walked upon the earth. Yet today and for all eternity he is exalted above all others. And he promises this to us as well. Remember his promises to you as you serve a person who may never thank you or even realize how much you do for them. You are following your Savior and you can take heart in the faithfulness you show in providing care for those who are vulnerable. You don't need to be ashamed of the things you do for another. You can rejoice in your lowly position, knowing what God has promised.

One caregiver, referring to Jesus' acts of humble service, told me, "If my Lord, who spoke this world into existence, was not above washing the feet of his followers, I can follow him by bathing Mom and wiping the food she dribbles." Providing care for someone with dementia probably wasn't in your future plans. Most likely, it interferes with other things you want or need to do: working at your job, taking care of your children, spending time with

> If you find yourself feeling burdened, worn out, discouraged, or even humiliated by the tasks you've taken on as a caregiver, remember the example of Christ. . . . You are following your Savior and you can take heart in the faithfulness you show in providing care for those who are vulnerable.

your spouse, or even doing things that you enjoy. When you become a caregiver, you sacrifice aspects of yourself to give to another. But remember this: God may have interrupted your plans to teach and form you into the person he wants you to be. He interrupts our lives for reasons we don't always understand. What seem to us to be frustrations and irritations can actually be the work of God, molding and shaping us into the image of Christ. The words of Dietrich Bonhoeffer are particularly appropriate as we think about the humility needed to serve others: "Nobody is too good for the lowest service.... We must be ready to allow ourselves to be interrupted by God, who will thwart our plans and frustrate our ways time and again, even daily, by sending people across our path with their demands and requests."[2]

So what might God be teaching us? How does he form us through the experience of caregiving?

We Need the Lord

My soul is weary with sorrow;
   strengthen me according to your word. (Psalm 119:28)

While it's good to follow Christ's example of sacrificial love, please know that you cannot do this alone — you need the Lord *and* the people he has placed around you to help you on this journey. Yes, you are called to follow Christ's example, but you are called to be a caregiver, *not* a savior. Christ does not have limits, but you do.

Learn what it means to lean heavily on the Lord. Bring him your needs and your failings, and he will listen. He will work his power through you. God tells us that his grace is sufficient for us, and when we feel weak we must remember that his power is made perfect in weakness (2 Corinthians 12:9). If we simply try harder, trusting in our own resources, wisdom, and strength, caregiving can feel like living in a dry and parched land. Keep in mind the warning of Jeremiah:

Cursed is the one who trusts in man,
   who draws strength from mere flesh
   and whose heart turns away from the LORD.

That person will be like a bush in the wastelands;
they will not see prosperity when it comes.
They will dwell in the parched places of the desert,
in a salt land where no one lives. (Jeremiah 17:5–6)

When we trust in our own strength, we eventually find that our well has run dry. There is nothing there to sustain us. We can get by for a time, but eventually we will be depleted. When our hearts turn away from the Lord as the source of our strength and hope, we become like a "bush in the wastelands." You may feel spiritually and emotionally parched, with nothing left to give. You haven't slept. You haven't had a moment of peace, and everything around you may seem to be crumbling. The person you take care of, who was once a source of joy and comfort, now seems to be doing everything to make your life difficult. What can you do? Where can you turn?

But blessed is the one who trusts in the LORD,
whose confidence is in him.
They will be like a tree planted by the water
that sends out its roots by the stream.
It does not fear when heat comes;
its leaves are always green.
It has no worries in a year of drought
and never fails to bear fruit. (Jeremiah 17:7–8)

When our trust is in the Lord we become like a tree sinking its roots deep below the surface into streams of living water. Sometimes we mistakenly think this means "looking on the bright side" or telling ourselves that things really aren't all that bad. But it is a mistake to deny the reality of suffering and pain. The Bible recognizes that there is suffering. Psalmists and prophets cry out in the Bible, and we can learn from them and seek to connect our experience with theirs. More than a third of the psalms are about crying out to God in trouble and distress; lament and faith complement one another.[3] They teach us that by trusting in the Lord and his provision we can continue to bear fruit, even though there may be drought all around us.

Trusting the Lord for Today

A caregiver I met shared with me the story from 1 Kings 17 as a way of thinking about God's provision in caregiving. In this passage, we meet Elijah, who has been living through a time of drought in the land. God instructs him to live in a ravine near the Jordan River, where he drinks from a brook and is fed by ravens. God provides for Elijah's needs, but eventually the brook dries up. So things look hopeless for Elijah, but God does not leave him there to die. Instead, God instructs him to leave for a nearby town where he will find a widow who will provide him with food. A hopeful promise, to be sure!

But when Elijah finds the widow she is far from hopeful:

> "As surely as the LORD your God lives," she replied, "I don't have any bread—only a handful of flour in a jar and a little olive oil in a jug. I am gathering a few sticks to take home and make a meal for myself and my son, that we may eat it—and die." (v. 12)

The picture is bleak. You sense that this woman has nothing left to give. Perhaps she has grown bitter, thinking the end has arrived. But the story doesn't end here. God supplies our needs, even when we are weak and depleted, so that we can give and provide for the needs of others. The story continues with Elijah's faithful response. He has heard God's promise to take care of him:

> Elijah said to her, "Don't be afraid. Go home and do as you have said. But first make a small loaf of bread for me from what you have and bring it to me, and then make something for yourself and your son. For this is what the LORD, the God of Israel, says: 'The jar of flour will not be used up and the jug of oil will not run dry until the day the LORD sends rain on the land.'" (v. 13–14)

The woman pushes past the breaking point and obeys, serving the prophet. And from this moment forward she finds that she always has enough—the flour is not used up and the oil does not run dry. Not only does she have enough to provide for herself and her son, she has enough for Elijah as well, in keeping with the word of the Lord (v. 16).

Each day God gives us what we need, even though it sometimes feels as though there is nothing left. As a caregiver, you can identify with this feeling. Today may have left you depleted, with nothing left. How will you possibly face tomorrow?

> *I remember my affliction and my wandering,*
> *the bitterness and the gall.*
> *I well remember them,*
> *and my soul is downcast within me.*
> *Yet this I call to mind*
> *and therefore I have hope:*
> *Because of the LORD's great love we are not consumed,*
> *for his compassions never fail.*
> *They are new every morning;*
> *great is your faithfulness.*
> *I say to myself, "The LORD is my portion;*
> *therefore I will wait for him." (Lamentations 3:19–24)*

Know that God's grace is new every morning. He always provides what we need and we must learn to wait on him. Sometimes God brings us to the end of ourselves so that our only option is to trust in him and bring our burdens to him.

Many caregivers worry about what will happen next: How long will I be able to care for my wife at home? Will we need to put Dad in a nursing home? How long will she be able to dress herself? Will my husband eventually forget who I am? As you struggle with the pain and uncertainty of these questions, call to mind the words of Jesus: "Do not worry about tomorrow, for tomorrow will worry about itself. Each day has enough trouble of its own" (Matthew 6:34). We don't know what tomorrow holds, and we cannot solve tomorrow's problems. When the Israelites were in the desert, God provided manna only one day at a time, and they

> How long will I be able to care for my wife at home? Will we need to put Dad in a nursing home? How long will she be able to dress herself? Will my husband eventually forget who I am?

were not to store up any for the next day.[4] They needed to learn to trust him to provide each day. Instead of worrying about things that no one can know or predict, we must also learn to trust his provision for us today. Jesus is calling to you to bring your worries, your weariness, and your burdens to him, so that you can find rest.

> Come to me, all you who are weary and burdened, and I will give you rest. Take my yoke upon you and learn from me, for I am gentle and humble in heart, and you will find rest for your souls. For my yoke is easy and my burden is light. (Matthew 11:28–30)

Be Still before the Lord

The Spirit draws us back to the Lord so that we find grace and rest in him. In the busyness of life we fail to remember God, but when we choose to "be still and know that [he is] God" (Psalm 46:10) we find peace and reassurance. Caregiving can become so task oriented that we forget the person we are serving. This can also happen in our walk with the Lord. We also become so task oriented that we forget to sit at our Savior's feet to rest in the presence of God.

> As Jesus and his disciples were on their way, he came to a village where a woman named Martha opened her home to him. She had a sister called Mary, who sat at the Lord's feet listening to what he said. But Martha was distracted by all the preparations that had to be made. She came to him and asked, "Lord, don't you care that my sister has left me to do the work by myself? Tell her to help me!"
>
> "Martha, Martha," the Lord answered, "you are worried and upset about many things, but few things are needed—or indeed only one. Mary has chosen what is better, and it will not be taken away from her." (Luke 10:38–42)

Caregiving may seem like an endless task, but God calls you to be still and to be present with him, even if it is just a brief time set apart from your routine. You may not be able to find a consistent time to read your Bible and pray quietly before you start your day (as you may have done during the pre-caregiving days). Instead, you may need to work these thing into your new caregiving routine.

Take a moment to sit at your Savior's feet. Be reminded of his love and grace. Remind yourself of his provision and his promise to be present. Take the time, even if only for a moment. One caregiver described this as having "mini-vacations," times when she would take a few moments to appreciate something God had made or done — perhaps the view from the side of the road on the way to a doctor's appointment. Ann Voskamp, talking of her own experience in cultivating a heart of gratitude, says: "When I give thanks for the seemingly microscopic, I make a place for God to grow within me."[5] Maybe all you can manage is a whispered prayer between tasks, but the Lord is calling you to remember him, what he has done for you, and what he has promised. Bring your burdens to him.

Grow in Grace

God pursues us and cares for us, even when we don't understand what he is doing. This is God's radical grace. He never turns away from us, even when we seem to resist his plans.

Monica cares for her mother every day and night. She loves her mother and always has. They've had a great relationship over the years, but after her mother developed dementia, her personality changed. Her once gentle spirit is now irritable and controlling. Her mother's cognitive changes progressed to the point that she became unable to care for herself, and things became more difficult. Her mother began to resist Monica's attempts to care for her, especially personal hygiene and bathing. When her mother began to smell badly, Monica would try to bathe her, but her mother would refuse and even fight her off by yelling or slapping. Her mother couldn't understand what she needed and didn't see that Monica was doing all of this out of love, knowing what was truly best for her mother.

A person with moderate to severe dementia sometimes cannot recognize their need for help. When those who love them try to do what is best, they may resist and fight them off. This difficult dynamic should remind us of another relationship — our relationship with our Lord. We often fail to realize that what God is doing in our life is for our good. All we focus on is how unpleasant it feels. Like the person suffering dementia, the second forgetting, our spiritual forgetfulness, leaves us confused and unable to recognize the goodness of God's long-term plan. So when God's plan doesn't line up with our plans, we resist.

Just the fact that we don't understand doesn't change the underlying truth. The one who cares for us does it in love, knowing what is best for us. Romans 8 says: "We know that in all things God works for the good of those who love him, who have been called according to his purpose" (v. 28). Caregiving provides us with an opportunity to grow in grace. Think about how this time in your life fits in with God's redemptive work in you. Remember that God reached out to you in love and grace to rescue you, even when you did not reach out to him (Romans 5:8). Know that God continues to reach out to you now, to care for you, even when you don't understand. You may try to slap his hand away. But be glad that this does not deter him. His love is strong, and he will continue to care for you even when you don't ask for it.

Be reminded of this when, as a caregiver, you provide care for your loved one with dementia. Even when they cannot appreciate what you are doing, know that you are doing it in love, for the good of the person. They may try to resist your efforts, to push you away. In those moments, remember that this is exactly what we do with God. Remembering this inclines our hearts toward grace. This grace can surround your caregiving when the person becomes difficult, yells at you, or in some other way pulls away from you. Let the comfort of God's unfailing love fill you and drive you to do the same for your loved one. Let your caregiving efforts flow out of God's grace shown to you, not out of a sense of duty or obligation.[6]

Imagine for a moment: how might your efforts to care for a vulnerable parent or spouse be transformed by grace? How does thinking about things this way change the way you look at the person? How does it change your care techniques?

Ask the Lord to help you see the person with dementia as God sees them: not as a bunch of deficits, but as one of his children redeemed by the sacrifice of Christ.

A Caregiver, Not a Savior

Our sacrifices are limited, however, in what they can achieve. We serve others, but we are not saviors. There are limits to what we can do. We can follow Christ's example to love in sacrificial service, but we do not have his ability to save people from sin. Sadly, our best caregiving efforts will not heal the person or prevent them from suffering, nor can we save them from the decline they will experience. Caregiving highlights our insufficiency. We can't do it all. In fact, there is only one sacrifice that is sufficient.

I've met many caregivers over the years. I recall one woman who had learned this lesson: her own efforts were not enough. She was quick to acknowledge she was not sufficient for this job because she would "crack, break, and crumble" if she relied only upon herself. "I tried to be perfect. But I need to pull back sometimes," she said. "I'm not God." Although she is her husband's caregiver, she is not his savior. But rather than despairing in her limits, she sees this as part of a journey that God has for her. "We are all in process ... sometimes we have to stand back and watch the Potter do his thing" (see Isaiah 64:8). The Lord works through our limitations to mold us as part of his redemptive plan for our lives.

Sacrifice can be good and loving, but we need to recognize when we are doing too much. Caregivers need to practice self-care, and they need to accept care from others. You are a key source of health, well-being, and spiritual support for your loved one. Outside of Christ, you are the most important person in their life right now. And although your sacrificial love is a beautiful expression of the gospel and Christ working in you, part of this involves allowing yourself to be cared for. Many caregivers fail to recognize their own need for care. Still others refuse to receive it, thinking that they need to focus only on their loved one with dementia. Caregivers who ignore or neglect their own health put themselves and their care recipient at risk. Caregivers who are highly stressed are at greater risk for depression. Research even suggests that the immune systems of highly stressed caregivers are weakened.[7] This means it is essential that you not wear yourself out.

One caregiver shared with me that like many with Alzheimer's disease, her husband began to develop a habit of repeating himself. This often adds to the stress felt by caregivers, but in this case it didn't. One of the things he would repeatedly say was, "I don't know what I would do without you." And, of course, he was right. His wife had taken on so much of his personal care, taking care of their home and finances, that if she were gone, he would be in trouble.

> One of the things he would repeatedly say was, "I don't know what I would do without you."

Some caregivers feel guilty about their need to be cared for, but consider this: you are *worth* taking care of. You matter to God—not in the abstract, but as a specific individual. Sacrificial love is good, but you cannot do it alone. Do your best, reach out to others, and put your hope in Christ and his provision.

Ministry to One

One caregiver wrote, "One morning as I awakened, I heard, 'Some minister to thousands and some minister to one.' I instinctively knew that familiar still small voice of the Holy Spirit. He was telling me that my life and service unto the Lord and my loved one was significant."[8] Indeed she is right. Consider the words of Jesus in Matthew 25:

> Then the King will say to those on his right, "Come, you who are blessed by my Father; take your inheritance, the kingdom prepared for you since the creation of the world. For I was hungry and you gave me something to eat, I was thirsty and you gave me something to drink, I was a stranger and you invited me in, I needed clothes and you clothed me, I was sick and you looked after me, I was in prison and you came to visit me."
>
> Then the righteous will answer him, "Lord, when did we see you hungry and feed you, or thirsty and give you something to drink? When did we see you a stranger and invite you in, or needing clothes and clothe you? When did we see you sick or in prison and go to visit you?"

The King will reply, "Truly I tell you, whatever you did for one of the least of these brothers and sisters of mine, you did for me." (vv. 34–40)

What might the Savior of your life say when you stand before him?

When I was forgetful, you remembered for me.
You answered my anxious questions even though I had asked them many times already.
When I was lost, you helped me find my way.
You helped take care of my money and gave me my medications when I couldn't.
When I lost my judgment, you kept me safe.
You even changed my clothes and helped me bathe.

"Truly I tell you, whatever you did for one of the least of these brothers and sisters of mine, you did for me."

FOR FURTHER REFLECTION

In this chapter we learned about God's grace in caregiving. Christ is the perfect caregiver and we are called to trust in his provision and imitate his example.

- How might God be using your caregiving experiences to grow your faith and to draw you closer to him? How might today's challenges be part of the longer redemptive journey God has for you?

- How can Christ's model of humble, sacrificial service influence the way you approach caregiving?

- If you aren't a caregiver, how can you encourage a caregiver to follow Christ's example of sacrificial love? How can you help them avoid trying to become a savior?

Chapter 7

ALZHEIMER'S
AND THE CHURCH

Adeline has been a follower of Christ for decades and has been in a nursing home for two long years. She is not happy there. She gets confused about where she is, often tries to leave, and sometimes yells at or hits those who get in her way. She doesn't often remember her children when they visit, and she sometimes seems to forget her husband of fifty years.

Her children long for someone to minister to her. The God-fearing mother they grew up with seems gone now, and her husband leaves his visits with her feeling hopeless. The pastor of their church wishes he could minister to her but doesn't see how. Adeline is confused and doesn't recognize him either. Even the nurses seem exasperated by her behavior. Nothing in the pastor's seminary training prepared him to deal with this.

The women from Adeline's Bible study visited her once, but they felt it did more harm than good. They asked her if she remembered them, which upset her. They asked her whether she liked the nursing home. She mumbled something they couldn't understand. They left feeling unsettled and worried, but soon their own challenges and the daily routine of life resumed, and they did not think of Adeline again. Each day, Adeline sits alone, and each night she lies down alone. Her isolation is broken only by the regular checks from the nursing staff. Her husband struggles as well. He longs for someone to step into his struggle to care for his wife, to help them keep their eyes focused on God.

For many reasons, the church at large has been absent in speaking about the struggle with Alzheimer's disease. The psychological components of Alzheimer's can frighten pastors and the general church body. After all, how can you minister to a person who doesn't remember who you are, who doesn't appear to understand what you're saying? It hardly seems worth the time when they won't even remember your visit. Many pastors feel ill-equipped to address the needs of people with dementia.

Most church communities look to their pastors for care in times of crisis. But the Bible doesn't leave this responsibility in the hands of a few. It expects the entire church to care for one another, not just the paid pastors and staff. This task of ministering to people affected by Alzheimer's and to their families is a church-wide responsibility. Unfortunately, those same feelings of fear and confusion keep individuals in the church from reaching out to those affected. The church needs help. We need to better equip people to minister, to overcome their lack of understanding, and to face their fears.

But another factor comes into play here as well. As one pastor said: "The church has an Alzheimer's of its own." Just as those with Alzheimer's are prone to forget things, the church is prone to forget those who aren't involved, who don't attend services or contribute in some way. When people are no longer present at church, they tend to be forgotten by pastors and church members alike. People get busy—out of sight, out of mind. In the very times when they are most in need, feeling isolated and alone, we tend to forget people with Alzheimer's.

Alzheimer's in My Church?

At first, you might be tempted to think that Alzheimer's is not an issue in your church. Perhaps not many people in the congregation have it. You may look around on Sunday morning and not notice anyone with Alzheimer's and assume it's not an issue you need to address. But this can be deceiving.

If you have an aging congregation, consider that 14 percent people over the age of seventy have dementia, and another 22 percent have some other form of cognitive impairment.[1] That means 36 percent of older people in your church are likely to have some form of significant cognitive decline. If you don't have many older adults in your church, you may still have a large number of baby boomers (those born between 1945 and 1964) who may be spending a good portion of their retirement either caring for a parent with Alzheimer's disease or who soon will develop the condition themselves. Some will have the experience of being both a caregiver and care recipient. In a recent report, the Alzheimer's Association described Alzheimer's as the "defining disease of the Baby Boom generation" and estimate that as many as ten million baby boomers will develop Alzheimer's disease.[2] At least that many will care for someone with the disease, if they haven't already.

People in the early stages of dementia will not stand out or appear much different in casual conversations after church. Many will be reluctant to share what is happening to them out of embarrassment or fear. Most people with Alzheimer's disease simply stop going to church. Some lack the initiative to get up on Sunday morning. Others lose their ability to drive and have no one to take them. Sometimes caregivers will be hesitant to bring their loved ones to church for fear they will do or say something inappropriate. But the fact that a person is absent from gatherings on Sunday mornings does not mean they are no longer part of the church.

The church is not a building or even a once-a-week gathering; it is a body of believers living and journeying together, bound to one another by faith in Christ. Some have made a distinction between the "gathered" church and the "scattered" church.[3] When the church gathers together each week, it is a time of learning, sharing community, and worship—but it is also a time for remembering.[4] The church can do many things when it gathers each week to welcome and minister to those with Alzheimer's. Yet even when a person can no longer attend the gatherings at the church building, the church body can do a lot for the "scattered." This chapter addresses how we can bring the church to families affected by dementia in practical and meaningful ways, both when we gather and when we are scattered.

So how can the church make a difference in caring for those with Alzheimer's? Some may ask, isn't this a medical problem with medical solutions? As we've seen, there are no cures, and families affected are left on their own as the person they love progressively declines. The church can help in the following ways:

- Offer physical, emotional, and spiritual support
- Help the person maintain as much independence as possible
- Help the person and their caregivers maintain a connection to the church body

Although church communities should be a natural place for people to turn in their suffering, the reality is that many don't. When the challenges of Alzheimer's first begin, many families lose touch with their church family or pastors. It is easy and all too common to turn on the church and criticize its failures, but let us not forget that a church is made up of sinners tied together by their desperate need of a Savior. Because it is filled with sinful human beings, the church does not have it all together. It will fail at times. You may feel like the church has let you down. That happens sometimes.

But that's not *all* the church is, by the grace of God. Under the guidance of the Holy Spirit, God is in the process of redeeming sinners and transforming lives. One pastor noted that instead of lamenting our failures, we should recognize the great opportunities before us in ministering to people affected by Alzheimer's and to their families. In these opportunities we can learn about faith, remembering, and grace. Churches may have forgotten people suffering through Alzheimer's in the past, but others are now seeing a divine opportunity to remember them and care for them. When this happens, God's glory is seen in a unique and beautiful way.

A community formed by the gospel has the potential to transform Alzheimer's care. When the church is healthy and aware of the good news of Jesus, they are more likely to be sacrificially involved in one another's lives. When troubles and sickness arise, brothers and sisters from the church can step in more naturally, and the person will be less likely to fade away from the church community. As the community surrounds the individual and their family, they can better understand their needs and ask pastors to step into the situation to help maintain that relationship.

The pastors and the members of the church body represent a tangible connection to God for the person struggling with Alzheimer's. We minister to people on God's behalf, and we pray to God on behalf of those we care for. In all of this, we look for unique opportunities to illustrate the gospel to the person, their caregivers, and anyone else who might be involved. As the church we should ask whether we as the body of Christ are reflecting our head, Jesus Christ. Jesus spent time with, touched, and ate with people whom the religious establishment of the day tended to avoid and shun. These people were isolated and marginalized, much like people with dementia are in today's culture.[5] Will today's church follow the lead of Jesus? Will we pursue those with dementia and embrace them like Jesus did the outcasts of his day?

Be an Advocate

One of the ways that the church can help is by being an advocate for people with Alzheimer's and their caregivers. What does that mean?

In John 14, Jesus tells his disciples that he is going away and they will not see him anymore. This sounds like bad news to them, but it is mixed with the good news of a promise that he is coming back, along with the hope of restoration. And Jesus offers them another promise as well—that he will send his Holy Spirit to serve a unique role in their lives. The Holy Spirit will provide guidance, comfort, and advocacy—serving as a mediator between God and man. Here Jesus describes the Holy Spirit with the word *Paraclete*, which can be interpreted as "one who comes alongside." Jesus refers to the Holy Spirit as an advocate and tells the disciples that the Holy Spirit will help them remember him and all that he has taught them.

All this I have spoken while still with you. But the Advocate, the Holy Spirit, whom the Father will send in my name, will teach you all things and will remind you of everything I have said to you. Peace I leave with you; my peace I give you. I do not give to you as the world gives. Do not let your hearts be troubled and do not be afraid. (John 14:25–27)

The Father sends the Holy Spirit to the disciples to remind them of his words so that they can be faithfully recorded for our benefit. Although this passage primarily refers to the origins of Scripture, attesting to its origin through the Holy Spirit,[6] it should also lead us to consider the role the Spirit has as an advocate today. The Spirit bears witness to the gospel so that we too can testify (John 15:26). The Spirit assures us of our enduring connection to the Father (Romans 8:15–16) and helps us understand the Word of God and the gospel (1 Corinthians 2:10–16), providing guidance in life and peace (Romans 8:4–8).[7]

This serves as a guide for how the church can care for families affected by Alzheimer's disease. Just as the Holy Spirit strengthens and builds up the church, we can, under the guidance of the Spirit, take on the role of a *paraclete*—an advocate. This includes coming alongside a family to help provide comfort, praying with them, mourning with them, and sometimes laughing with them. People need advocacy that helps them to connect with the church body and mobilize resources for them. They need guidance in coping with Alzheimer's disease and remembering the Lord.

Be Willing to Journey

It is not good for people with Alzheimer's to be alone. It is also not good for caregivers to try to do everything on their own. Alzheimer's brings people to the end of themselves and shows their limits in ways they may have never imagined. They need the strength of the Lord, his wisdom, and his grace. They also need to be surrounded with a caring community.

Many caregivers are reluctant to ask for help. Some feel guilty leaving their loved one with someone else because they believe they should be able to provide for all of the person's needs on their own. Others may have a sense of shame or embarrassment over the person's condition or in their inability to go it alone. Still others believe that getting help is not worth the time and effort it takes to get other people to understand their situation and the person they care for.

> We need to remember that we minister to people not in hopes of halting the disease but to encourage their trust in God and to experience the love he has for us.

Even though the church can be a source of comfort and help, many stop going to church and are hesitant to share their needs. As a result, pastors and individuals within the church may need to take the initiative. The church has great potential in ministering to people with Alzheimer's, but how to begin is not always obvious. Alzheimer's is confusing. It's hard to know how to communicate, to step in, and to feel as if you are really making a difference because the sad truth is that the underlying progression of the disease will march on, no matter what you do. We need to remember that we minister to people not in hopes of halting the disease but to encourage their trust in God and to experience the love he has for us. Alzheimer's dims a person's outlook. So the role of the church community is to step in and throw open the windows to let the light of hope shine in.

The first step to take is simply to be present. Don't pull back from relationships with these individuals and families.[8] Journey with your brothers and sisters during this time. One woman wrote to me:

> Mother was a true servant in the church for over sixty years. Dad was a trustee, sang in the choir. As their ability to participate lessened, they were forgotten. It felt like—if they couldn't serve the church, the church moved on to people who could. A few close friends offered to have Dad for lunch so Mother could go to a doctor's appointment without taking him, but there was no church involvement to support or help her. They didn't even visit. Ironically, one of her functions in her early eighties

was to coordinate care for people in need within the church. A few short years later, when she was in need, nobody came. As she became less able to interact socially, even the occasional phone call ceased. One longtime friend from church called me to ask how she was. She admitted that she never called Mother anymore because she wasn't sure Mother knew who she was or remembered the call. I encouraged her to call, identify herself, and just share what was going on in her life—that Mother would love hearing from her even if just for the time of the call. It disappoints me a great deal that when it came "her turn," no one from the church stepped up to the plate.

People long for loving connections with those in the church body. One wife I talked with longed for someone to connect with her, but even more, she longed for someone to take an interest in and spend time connecting with her husband, a former missionary who now suffers with Alzheimer's:

He needs male companionship ... to have one or two men to visit him and show an interest in him (who he was, and who he is), and perhaps even take him for a short ride or something. Give him time with trusted friends who understand his situation and don't always ask questions needing an answer, and who speak slowly, and articulate clearly, and aren't in a hurry. Men who will pray with him, and know how to talk about something other than sports or politics or business. Men who can affirm his accomplishments and contributions, and give him respect. Men who care! I would rather have someone minister to him than to try to meet my needs. I'll manage, but time is slipping away from him.

When I interview caregivers and ask what the church can do for them, the most common response is: They simply want the church to be present in their lives through the journey of dementia. They do not want to be alone.

Caregivers who care for a spouse with dementia experience aloneness. The relationship they once had with their loving spouse now feels like it's gone. As she sits with her husband in the "golden years" of retirement, the space that was once filled with conversation and laughter is now filled with an oppressive silence. He stares straight ahead, not speaking. It isn't that he is unable to speak—if you work at it and engage him, he will respond. He is still there, but he has changed. She loves him as she always has, and her covenant commitment to him has not diminished. It is a beautiful testimony, yes. But she is *lonely*. Her companion feels far away, even as he sits next to her.

It is obvious that she cannot leave him alone. It would be a safety risk. But the truth we often miss is that we cannot leave *her* alone either. To be present, to care for families like this, we must go to them, we must initiate. The church should take initiative by pursuing these families in love. We must move toward them, just as Christ did for us (1 John 4:19; Romans 5:8).

> They simply want the church to be present in their lives through the journey of dementia. They do not want to be alone.

Gospel community can come to a person's home in the form of a small group or community group. Even if the person doesn't contribute much to the discussion, they are still present with others in the body of Christ. If the person lives in a nursing home or another long-term-care setting, a group could meet in the community room or multipurpose space. Bring the kids and make it a multigenerational experience. Many people with Alzheimer's light up when children are present (although there are exceptions as well).

Because Alzheimer's is such a complex disease, people tend to think that our approaches to helping must also be complex. But when Jesus speaks about what we can do for him and "the least of these," the things he mentions are pretty simple. Bring food to a hungry person. Invite a stranger in. Visit the sick. The first step is to be present in suffering and uncertainty. When we step in and remain present, we communicate love and a willingness to bear one another's burdens. Our presence speaks louder than our words. In 1 John 4:10–12, we learn how we can respond to God's love for us by loving one another:

> This is love: not that we loved God, but that he loved us and sent his Son as an atoning sacrifice for our sins. Dear friends, since God so loved us, we also ought to love one another. No one has ever seen God; but if we love one another, God lives in us and his love is made complete in us.

By being present with those who are hurting and confused, we become a concrete reminder that God is present. We come alongside families and journey with them, encouraging and supporting them, and demonstrating the love of Christ in a practical way. One practical aspect of this is that we get to know the person and their caregivers better and more appropriately begin to address whatever needs arise. You don't need to know all of the right things to say. Just be present. Be quick to listen and slow to speak (James 1:19). Weep with those who weep and mourn with those who mourn (Romans 12:15).

Job's three friends come to him when they hear about his great troubles.

> When [they] heard about all the troubles that had come upon him, they set out from their homes and met together by agreement to go and sympathize with him and comfort him. When they saw him from a distance, they could hardly recognize him; they began to weep aloud, and they tore their robes and sprinkled dust on their heads. Then they sat on the ground with him for seven days and seven nights. No one said a word to him, because they saw how great his suffering was. (Job 2:11–13)

Job's friends get it right—until they open their mouths to speak. But their first response, to go to their friend, to be with him in his suffering, and to just be present out of love and compassion, is one that we can learn from. They came to sit with Job and mourn with him after he lost everything but God. We too can sit and mourn with those who have lost so much to Alzheimer's. And we can help them remember that they have not lost God.

Address Practical Needs

The demands of providing full-time care take a toll. Caregivers need time to rest, to take care of other aspects of life, and to be still and enjoy friendships. If you haven't been a caregiver, it is difficult to understand how little spare time they have. In addition to being present with them, you can give the gift of time as well.

Respite and Rest

Providing a caregiver with time away from the demands of caregiving is like giving them a cup of cool water. This time can free them up and change their outlook on their situation—allowing them to provide better care when they return. In this way, your gift of time allows the caregiver to extend grace to the person with Alzheimer's.

Unfortunately, this is not as easy as just stepping in, unless you've known the person for some time. The caregiver and the person with Alzheimer's both need to feel comfortable with you.

If you've ever been responsible for the care of other people, you know how important it is to have someone you trust watch over things while you are away. But you need more than trust. That person needs to be familiar with the people and tasks they are watching over; otherwise they won't know what to do if problems arise. If you're a parent, for instance, a regular sitter will already be so familiar with your kids that they won't need to be told about the unique concerns with each child. This reduces your anxiety. You can relax and not worry when you go away. What if you were to become that person, getting to know the person with Alzheimer's so well that the caregiver could relax and feel comfortable leaving them alone with you?

Get to know the person they care for. Encourage them to tell you their story. Listen in love, with patience. Take the time to slow down and sit with the person to honor and love them by listening and encouraging them with your time and passages from the Word. Become an expert on that person. Many caregivers feel overwhelmed by the physical and emotional demands of providing care. It is a huge gift to them when you spend time with their loved one.

Caregivers also have emotional demands. Your willingness to step in and give them a break will alleviate some of the emotional burden they carry. They now have someone to walk alongside them, someone to talk with who really understands the subtleties of the person and their care. They have an empathetic person they can call when things get tough.

Help Around the Home

In addition to providing rest for caregivers, you can be an advocate for their practical needs. Some families need help with chores or taking care of things around the home. Some do not have time or energy to take care of their lawn. Others may not have the technical expertise or strength needed to make physical repairs to their home. Some need help moving things around inside the home. Others need help packing up for a difficult move to a nursing home. Imagine the physical and emotional difficulty of such a transition. This is an opportunity to be emotionally and spiritually present, while assisting with physical tasks.

In 1 John 3:16–18, we read that we should imitate the love of Christ by caring for the practical, physical needs of people:

> This is how we know what love is: Jesus Christ laid down his life for us. And we ought to lay down our lives for our brothers and sisters. If anyone has material possessions and sees a brother or sister in need but has no pity on them, how can the love of God be in that person? Dear children, let us not love with words or speech but with actions and in truth.

Some caregivers would be greatly blessed if you would pick up their groceries for them. Others would prefer to have someone stay in their home while they got out of the house themselves to buy the groceries. Making a meal provides the caregiver with some rest in an otherwise busy routine. As you get to know the family and their situation, you will be able to identify their practical needs and recruit others to help.

Financial Help

Caregivers also have financial burdens. The costs of providing care have skyrocketed, and many caregivers have to give up their jobs to provide care. Fifty-six percent of families report that Alzheimer's caused a financial strain for many families. Pray about how you can help a family with everyday provisions: bringing in meals, picking up the tab at the grocery, or, if you are financially able, helping to pay for healthcare needs.

One woman who had developed dementia still loved to be active by exercising and biking. Her husband dutifully brought her to an exercise facility regularly several times each week. As her dementia advanced, he was unable to get her there even though this was an important part of her routine and a key part of her physical and emotional well-being. Their church saw a need and stepped in by providing her with a stationary bike that she could ride at home. She continued to ride it for miles each day. Given their medical costs, the family was unlikely to purchase this on their own, but the church sought to care for them through this gift.

Be creative! Pray for guidance, and base your service on what you know about the person and their family. Care should always be tailored to the individual and family.

Doctors' Appointments

Caregivers who drive themselves and their loved one to doctors' appointments in urban areas sometimes have to choose between parking far from the doctor's office and facing a long walk (which can be an issue) or dropping off their loved one with dementia at the door and hoping they won't wander off. Offer to help by dropping both the caregiver and the person with dementia off at the door while you park the car.

Visits to the doctor are also times when new information on the progress of the disease is shared—which is not often good news. Having someone present offers comfort and encouragement, and it can also help the caregiver later recall what the doctor said. When people feel overwhelmed, their memory can fail, whether dementia is an issue or not.

You can also offer to drop off or pick up the prescription afterward so they can go home and rest. Buy them lunch or coffee. For the person with dementia, sharing a good meal can be a concrete comfort that helps shift their mood after a difficult medical visit. Food won't make everything right, but having a pleasant event after these visits can go a long way toward helping them feel better.

Share the Gospel and Do Good

The church is called to cling to and remember the good news of the gospel—and to let it sink deeply into our hearts and minds. We remind each other that we have been rescued from our old identity of sin and death and have been delivered by grace alone into a new life in the Holy Spirit. This life is eternal and begins now, even as we still live in decaying bodies. Our true identity is not tied to these failing bodies, but to our life in Christ. Knowing this frees us, as a church, to live out our calling, devoting ourselves to two main things we can do for families with Alzheimer's. First, we should remind those who are suffering of the good news of the gospel. But in addition, we should do good works on behalf of the person and family affected by the disease. We do the latter *because of* the first. We are rescued and reborn in order that we can do good to others.

In reminding others of the good news of the gospel, we preach it to ourselves as well. When we teach others we will understand and integrate the truth more deeply. Integrating truth with concrete actions exhibits fruitful faith, as described in the book of James. This integration of knowledge and action makes us less prone to forget the gospel. By God's grace, as we seek to minister to others, we find that our own faith is strengthened.

Tips for Interacting
with People with Alzheimer's

Don't take it personally if the person can't remember your name. This is one of the hallmarks of the disease. Even if you feel like you really connected with the person before, it will not affect their ability to remember your name. If the person had the ability to remember your name, they would.

Don't ask them if they remember you or your name. They may remember you, just not your name. Asking them if they remember you puts them on the spot and can serve to highlight their deficits. You wouldn't ask a person with poor vision if they can see you or if they like your new shirt. Instead, just greet them by name and show genuine interest and enthusiasm to be with them. If you do, they will likely be glad for your presence even if they don't remember you or your name.

Don't quiz people about what they do and don't remember. If you want to talk about a shared memory you have with the person, it is better to say, "I remember the time we ..." If you begin talking about the event or memory, they may join in if they remember (and are interested). If you don't have shared experiences, use what you know of the person and begin by saying something like, "I heard you once [insert an accomplishment or event]" or "I understand that you like ..."

Don't be surprised if the person is glad to see you one day and doesn't seem to want you there the next. People with Alzheimer's are as affected by the everyday hassles of life as you are. If you didn't sleep well, or had an argument with your spouse, or were disappointed over something that didn't go right, it would affect your mood, your patience, and maybe even your desire to be around other people. People with Alzheimer's are affected by these things too, and sometimes to an even greater degree.

Don't try to convince them to see things the way you do. Sometimes people with dementia have beliefs or explanations for things that are incorrect (for instance, they think someone is stealing from them, or that they're still sixteen years old, or that their long-dead spouse is still living). These experiences are real for them, and you won't have much success convincing them they aren't true. Acknowledging that you've heard them and gently redirecting them to another topic will be much more effective.

Visit, but be flexible. Caregiving for someone with advancing dementia can be quite unpredictable. Something could come up that is out their control and they may need to cancel.

Keep the noise and activity level relatively low. Although this can vary, those with moderate to severe Alzheimer's disease are more easily overwhelmed by an overly busy or noisy environment. Their ability to handle stress decreases as the disease progresses, and therefore a stressful environment can lead to feelings of anxiety and agitated behavior.

Don't startle or surprise them. People with dementia startle easily. Get their attention by standing in front of them before you speak, if possible.

Do not talk to them as if they are children; remember they are adults. Many people draw comparisons between parenting a young child and caring for a person with advanced dementia (as I did above when discussing respite). As they lose the ability to care for themselves, they need others to do more for them and watch over them to keep them safe, just as a young child does. But remember that they deserve the honor and respect of an adult with decades of life experience and even wisdom. Speak to them as adults, and if they have trouble understanding, you can always adjust by speaking more slowly and with simpler language.

Avoid combining multiple ideas or requests into one statement. For example: "Why don't you have a seat over here where we can talk. I'd like to hear about your grandchildren. Do you want some tea?" would be less confusing if broken into three separate statements. After "Why don't you have a seat?" allow the person to sit down before asking if they want tea. After tea is served, then ask about their grandchildren.

Listen first, then listen some more. Not many people listen to what a person with dementia has to say. Not many ask them what they think, feel, or want. Take time to listen to what they have to say. Similarly, some caregivers have told me that people have tried to comfort them by telling them that others "have it worse" or that "things could be worse." This is not helpful. It is better to take time to understand what that person is experiencing and how they are coping with the challenges of caregiving.

- -

FOR FURTHER REFLECTION

In this chapter we learned several ways that the church can begin to step into the lives of people with dementia and their caregivers. Consider your church community or neighborhood and begin to pray about how you can be present with those who are suffering with dementia.

- How can you offer practical and spiritual support to the caregiver? The person with dementia?

- Pray that God will give the church a vision for caring for some of the most vulnerable people in today's society. What would it look like if they church looked for opportunities to share the love of Christ with this group of people?

- -

Chapter 8

REMEMBERING
STORIES OF FAITH

S TORYTELLING IS AN EASY TOOL TO USE with those suffering with
dementia. The simple act of remembering and discussing aspects
of one's story is usually enjoyable in itself. People feel good, laugh,
and sometimes cry when they recall positive events and relationships.
Such emotional responses are beneficial, and they can draw people
together, helping them feel comfort in the moment. People may also
grow quiet, weep, and even feel angry when they recall difficult times.
Retelling a difficult story can also help the person achieve some reso-
lution of a past conflict or gain some new understanding or insight.[1]
People like telling their stories regardless of whether some new understanding results. When people retell the stories of their lives they are
reminded of who they really are, where they came from, and what is
truly important.

The Power of Stories

It has been a long day for Raymond. The doctor's office has a funny smell and the lights feel too bright. He has been sitting in the same seat for quite some time, but he is unsure how long. A woman sitting across a table from him has been asking him questions that he hadn't anticipated.

"I'm going to read a list of words to you, and when I finish, I want you to tell me all the words that you can remember." After she finished reading the words, he struggled to recall a few, but it was clear to both of them that he had already forgotten much of it. His frustration was clear. It was embarrassing to be unable to remember something that he had just heard. His face was downcast, and he did not speak.

Then she asks him about his life, his work, and his family. His relief is obvious. As he begins to speak, his eyes light up. He becomes more expressive and finds himself laughing. He talks in great detail about raising his daughters and his work as a school teacher.

It is good to remember. It takes us back in time and helps us reexperience things we've gone through that helped define who we are. Sometimes the remembering and reexperiencing are prompted by a smell or a song, and we seem to be ushered back into another era.

Although remembering our individual stories is beneficial, we derive even greater benefit when we connect our story to the larger story of God. In Craig Bartholomew and Michael Goheen's book *The Drama of Scripture*, the authors explain that we only find meaning and true understanding of our stories when we understand them as part of the larger story of Scripture.[2] Remembering the Lord and his faithfulness on our journey is a central command of Scripture and one that helps root us in our identity as the people of God. Situating our individual stories within the gospel story provides comfort in times of suffering.

Each summer my family spends time on a small lake in Michigan. One of our kids' favorite activities is to swim off the pontoon boat at the far end of the lake. Their grand-

> When we tell stories and recall our faith journey, we anchor our lives more firmly to God's story.

father drives the boat across the lake, and when we reach the swimming spot, one of us lifts the anchor and drops it over the side. Once it catches the bottom, the anchor is out of sight, hidden deep below the surface. We don't pay much attention to it until the winds come. If the rope has some slack, the wind will blow our boat for a short distance, but eventually the anchor does its job. The rope pulls tight, yanking the boat back as it catches.

An anchor works below the surface. It keeps the boat from drifting away no matter what storms may come. Much like an anchor, God gives us his promise to anchor our lives so we do not drift, especially when the storms of life threaten to capsize us (Hebrews 6:19). When we tell our stories, we need to anchor the boat of our lives to something solid—and what could be more firm than the faithfulness and promises of God? When we tell stories and recall our faith journey, we anchor our lives more firmly to God's story.

> We don't always know what questions or old memories serve as effective identity anchors. We may need to explore a bit, much like we sometimes need to drop an anchor in more than one location to find the spot where it will catch and hold.

One caregiver told me that reviewing her life story helped her to understand how some of the most difficult events in her early life had prepared her to care for her husband, who was plagued with an atypical form of dementia. "Everything I've learned and gone through has led me here and enabled me to care for him." She had lost her mother at an early age and had been forced to step in and take care of others in her family as a young child. Although this was painful, she now sees how this helped her develop the skills that she now needs. Even more importantly, it taught her how to persevere, trusting in the Lord through the difficult aspects of caregiving. The gospel provided her with a framework, an anchor for understanding her experience from a deeper perspective.

When working with a person who has dementia, we don't always know what questions or old memories serve as effective identity anchors. We may need to explore a bit, much like we sometimes need to drop an anchor in more than one location to find the spot where it will catch and hold. This can take time and may be frustrating at first, but patiently pursuing a person's story in love is a way of honoring them.

> **What matters is honoring their desire to be heard and understood.**

Learning to Listen

You will find that people with Alzheimer's tell their stories in a different way than other people do. Their stories may not follow a strict linear progression. They may be repetitive and may not make sense at first. You may need to work at this, just as you would with a piece of literature or a symbolic film. You may not be able to sit back and let the story come to you. You will need to work at listening, piecing together fragmented parts to better understand.

Keep in mind that the goal of listening is not only hearing what the person has said, but also what he has *tried* to say.[3] The person may be confused as they speak. If what the person says isn't clear, ask yourself, "What did he or she mean to say? How does this fit with what he has said before? How does this connect with what I know about him?"

Again, there may be a lot of repetition, and that can be frustrating. But repetition can also be a clue. It may mean that this aspect of the story is important or has emotional significance. On the other hand, it may just be something the person is stuck on. When the person tells their story, you can honor them by letting the repetition go rather than telling them that they've already told you this before.

Honoring Parents

The Scriptures command us to honor our fathers and mothers, yet for many caregiving children this is a tricky task. How do you honor your father or mother when the roles have been reversed, when it is the child now taking care of the parent? Let me suggest several ways:

- Take the time to listen
- Make an effort to understand despite confusion
- Be patient with repetition
- Take the initiative in helping them remember and tell their story
- Do not point out their memory failure

Research has demonstrated that people with dementia can engage in a form of life review with the assistance of another caring person. This has been shown to be beneficial in reducing distress and achieving other positive outcomes.[4] However, the application of life review techniques has not yet been applied to telling and rehearsing one's story of faith, at least in the context of Alzheimer's research. In other words, the research doesn't offer us much guidance. It doesn't tell us what aspects of the story are most important. This means that we should explore a variety of stories with people. People with dementia should be encouraged to discuss significant events from earlier parts of their life, spiritual struggles they have had, important relationships, things for which they are grateful, as well as regrets and confessions.

Since people with Alzheimer's disease can be confused about time and place, it's not as important that the time sequence is correct. What matters is honoring their desire to be heard and understood. If a person confuses the order of events or seems to have something out of place, show them grace by letting it go. Listen for important themes, events, and struggles, and ignore the cognitive problems that may make them feel ashamed or embarrassed.

We can also use Bible stories or meaningful elements of a person's faith to help them. Well-known Scripture passages and hymns can help the person remember who God is and what he has promised. Consistent with some of the research done on spirituality in those with Alzheimer's, multisensory stimuli can be used to assist in this process.[5] Smells, sounds, and sights can prompt recollection of different parts of a person's story. Pictures and music can be particularly helpful for people with memory impairment.

Rose was taking care of her husband who had many health problems. Not only had she been his wife of sixty years, she was also his full-time caregiver. Generally, she managed the tasks well. Once in a while she would mix up his medications and sometimes seemed a little confused herself. Her family knew how demanding and stressful caregiving can be, and they didn't worry much about her memory and cognition. Eventually, her husband's body gave out, and he passed away. Losing a spouse of sixty years is a challenge for anyone, and this loss hit Rose harder than her children expected. She became more confused and forgetful. Her sleep patterns got out of sync. Before her husband became ill she had kept a tidy home where everything had its place. Now, things were scattered around the home. Even worse, the food and milk in the refrigerator had clearly gone bad.

Over the course of just a few months the caregiver had shifted to the receiving end, and her children were now caring for her. They prayed that things would improve, that this was just a temporary expression of grief. But as time went by, nothing improved. Eventually one of Rose's daughters had to quit her job to take care of her because she was afraid to leave her mother alone. Even though her mood improved over time, the forgetfulness and confusion remained. Her doctor suspected she had Alzheimer's.

It wasn't clear if Rose understood this or remembered when the initial diagnosis was made. Even as her care needs increased, she kept her friendly disposition and seemed generally content. She was well taken care of. Eventually, however, her care needs exceeded what the family could provide, and they made the decision to move her into a nursing home.

Packing up your parent's belongings to move into a nursing home can be incredibly difficult, particularly for those who have been care-givers to a parent. There is some relief at no longer having day-to-day, hour-to-hour, minute-to-minute responsibility for someone. On the other hand, great sadness and a sense of guilt can sometimes creep in. Some feel a sense of failure, thinking that if they had tried a little harder, given a little more, or sacrificed more of themselves, they could have prevented this from happening. But even our best efforts cannot save a person from Alzheimer's. Eventually things fall out of our control.

As her daughter was packing up and cleaning out Rose's things, she took the opportunity to review and learn more about her mother's life. She reconstructed some of Rose's life into the form of a book, a resource that would help Rose remember her journey, despite her confusion.

Her daughter found some old photos, her marriage certificate, and other important documents from various stages in her life. She also found several old prayers and poems that seemed to be meaningful to Rose. One of the poems was the "Prayer of St. Francis de Sales," which was especially fitting. It was familiar to Rose and it also seemed to speak to the uncertainty of her condition and the reality of her struggle.

Be at Peace
Do not look forward in fear to the changes of life;
rather look to them with full hope as they arise.
God, whose very own you are,
will deliver you from out of them.
He has kept you hitherto,
and He will lead you safely through all things;
and when you cannot stand it,
God will bury you in His arms.
Do not fear what may happen tomorrow;
the same everlasting Father who cares for you today
will take care of you then and every day.
He will either shield you from suffering,
or will give you unfailing strength to bear it.
Be at peace,
and put aside all anxious thoughts and imagination.

ST. FRANCIS DE SALES (1567–1622)

Rose took comfort in the book her daughter had created and used it to help her think back to earlier times. Her daughter saw the impact it had on her mother and began creating more books and using familiar prayers and Scripture passages, integrating them into cards with photos from earlier in life. She honored her mother by making sure the book was carefully constructed, artistically designed, and tailored to cover the details of Rose's long life.

Rose's positive experience with these books highlights several key aspects of our memory process. Each time Rose looked at the books, she was able to recognize the pictures and items, and she experienced great joy in doing so. Remarkably, each time she opened it was like seeing the book for the first time. Each time it felt like a brand-new gift from her daughter. The books provided her with concrete reminders to anchor her life and identity during a confusing and uncertain phase. Even when Rose seemed unable to tell her own story aloud, these books provided her with an opportunity to remember.

Her daughter also wrote down some comforting and well-known Bible passages and surrounded them with pictures of her mother with friends and relatives. This had the effect of drawing her attention to them and helping her see the verses. Her daughter had shown great honor for her mother, using Scripture passages that had been personally meaningful to her and connecting them with pictures that would be most likely to prompt her memory. The books also provided her with comfort in the midst of her suffering.

There is more than one way to help someone with Alzheimer's remember. Some people with Alzheimer's will want to tell their story over and over. The repetition is sometimes an attempt to hold on to some aspect of their identity and personhood. Other people with Alzheimer's may not speak but will listen as you recount stories from their life and speak of God's faithfulness, showing them pictures and objects from their past. You can't gauge the meaningfulness of these activities by the person's presence or lack of a response. We cannot fully know what is going on in the mind and heart of a person with more advanced Alzheimer's. But we can take comfort that the Holy Spirit is at work, reminding them of the Lord (Romans 8:14–17). Pray that the Lord will help them remember and allow you peace in trusting him even when the person doesn't show an obvious response.

Practical Steps for Getting Started

Avoid starting your time with the words, "Do you remember …" Instead, begin by talking about a general time period in their life and let them pick up as they are able. When a person has trouble telling their story or starting off, consider starting with an object or picture rather than a question. You could also start by talking about your own life, sharing your story with them, and letting them join in as they wish.

For the person with dementia, a mix of simple reminiscence and life review questions is the best strategy. Simple reminiscence encourages the person to share memories, whereas life review questions tend to focus on reflection and new insights to a greater degree. As the person progresses through dementia, the balance of prompts and questions will tip more toward reminiscence, but it is worth using both types — people with dementia can sometimes surprise you with what they remember.

Most forms of reminiscence and life review tend to be structured around life stages: childhood, adolescence, early adulthood, middle adulthood, and later life. Questions should touch on these broad stages, but are only starters. Learn to listen for key events and relationships in the person's life, and follow up on these with additional questions. By listening, you can piece together their story of faith so that you can then help them be reminded of the Lord and his faithfulness throughout their life.

It is also important to listen for spiritual concerns the person has, which you might be able to address either alone or with the assistance of a pastor.

A mix of questions, such as the following, about life in general and life of faith will yield the best results.[6]

- What was your life like as a child?

- What was your family like while you were growing up?

- Did you grow up in the church? What was your experience with church like as a child?
- Were you a good student?
- Tell me about your relationship with the Lord when you were younger.
- How is that relationship different (or the same) now?
- What are your thoughts on marriage? Raising children?
- Were there times when your faith in God helped you through difficulty?
- Tell me about your job.
- How did you decide to retire?
- When you look back on your life, what are you most thankful for?
- Who are some of the most important people in your life?
- Looking back over your life, what do you remember with joy?
- As you get older, what are you looking forward to?
- How has the church supported you (or not) as you've grown older?

Be patient. Take your time. Some questions may prompt remembering and others will seem to fail. Involve another family member or friend. Make this an enjoyable social remembrance.

These questions can be combined with the activities offered in chapter 9. Procedural and emotional aspects of memory are key — doing and feeling often prompt remembering.

Sharing Stories with Others Affected by Alzheimer's

When a person offers their testimony, they are essentially recounting their story of faith and offering concrete instances of how the gospel transformed their lives. Testimonies serve an important function in communities of faith. Recalling one's story in connection with God's larger story has a variety of positive benefits both to the teller and to the listener.

The book of Exodus tells how Moses' father-in-law, Jethro, visits him, and after greeting him, Moses recounts the story of God's faithfulness to him:

> Moses told his father-in-law all that the LORD had done to Pharaoh and to the Egyptians for Israel's sake, all the hardship that had befallen them on the journey, and *how* the LORD had delivered them. Jethro rejoiced over all the goodness which the LORD had done to Israel, in delivering them from the hand of the Egyptians. So Jethro said, "Blessed be the LORD who delivered you from the hand of the Egyptians and from the hand of Pharaoh, *and* who delivered the people from under the hand of the Egyptians. Now I know that the LORD is greater than all the gods ..." (Exodus 18:8–11 NASB)

Upon hearing about God's faithfulness, Jethro himself testifies to the greatness of God and is encouraged in his belief. We see that in addition to helping Moses and his people to remember, sharing stories of God's work can encourage the faith of others and lead us to celebrate God's grace and provision.

John Swinton explains that the dominant storyline of dementia is one of progressive decline, and it situates people almost exclusively in the context of disease, deficits, and death.[7] If we, as the people of God, fail to rehearse and share the stories of faith with those with Alzheimer's and other dementias, we are allow this depressing, hopeless story to remain the dominant narrative, leaving people without the expectation of hope, joy, and love in the later years of life. But if we testify about God's grace in the midst of these trials we give hope to others, even the next generation of people with dementia and their caregivers.

> *God is our refuge and strength,*
>   *an ever-present help in trouble.*
> *Therefore we will not fear, though the earth give way*
>   *and the mountains fall into the heart of the sea....*
> *The LORD Almighty is with us;*
>   *the God of Jacob is our fortress.*
> *Come and see what the LORD has done. (Psalm 46:1–2, 7–8)*

Even though the waters churn around us, our hope, identity, and refuge is in the finished work of Christ and the promises of God. This is our anchor. God help us to remember!

FOR FURTHER REFLECTION

Our stories matter — to us, to God, and to those he has placed around us. Remembering our stories and the ways God has led us has many benefits and can encourage our own faith and the faith of those around us.

- Take time to sit with someone and ask them to share some of their story with you.

- Take time to remember and review your story, and maybe even share it with someone you love and trust. As you do this, take notice of things that you end up writing or telling someone that you previously had seemed to forget. Are there parts of your journey that you hadn't thought about before this activity? Are there ways in which you have forgotten the Lord in your journey? How can you better remember this moving forward?

Chapter 9

REMEMBERING THE LORD

ALTHOUGH PEOPLE WITH ALZHEIMER'S DISEASE cannot remember some things, we might wrongly assume that they cannot remember anything. This is not true. They can remember many things using the memory systems that remain.[1]

The focus of this chapter is on ways to help us remember our faith in God and his faithfulness to us. We will look at how the essentials of the gospel can be rehearsed and remembered in a meaningful way through the combined use of the sacraments (such as Communion), well-known Scripture passages, music, and liturgy. We will focus on methods that are familiar, easy to incorporate, and that maximize understanding. These can inform how ministry leaders might modify their approach to compensate for the cognitive changes caused by Alzheimer's.

Our goal in ministering to those with Alzheimer's is to help them remember God's story and how their own story of faith is situated within that larger story of redemption. God calls us to himself to know him, to love him, and to experience his goodness and provision. He calls us to remember him for his glory and for our good.

When God calls us to remember him, he already knows we are prone to forget. Remembering God isn't easy for anyone, whether we have Alzheimer's or not. But God provides ways for us to recall who he is and what he has done. God uses several methods in Scripture to help us remember:

- Physical reminders
- Community-based remembering
- Reading and rehearsing Bible passages and stories
- Multisensory methods like music and Communion
- Prayer and the guidance of the Holy Spirit

Each of these methods help us to rehearse and remember the story of God. They are not specific to those with Alzheimer's disease and can benefit any believer who wants help remembering God.

Physical Reminders

God gives us physical reminders of what he has done and promised for his people. For example, before the Israelites crossed over into the Promised Land, God gave them instructions for how to remember this event and the story leading up to it.

> So Joshua called together the twelve men he had appointed from the Israelites, one from each tribe, and said to them, "Go over before the ark of the Lord your God into the middle of the Jordan. Each of you is to take up a stone on his shoulder, according to the number of the tribes of the Israelites, to serve as a sign among you. In the future, when your children ask you, 'What do these stones mean?' tell them that the flow of the Jordan was cut off before the ark of the covenant of the Lord. When it crossed the Jordan, the waters of the Jordan were cut off. These stones are to be a memorial to the people of Israel forever." (Joshua 4:4–7)

God instructed the people to pile up the rocks as reminders to those who laid them and to future generations of what he had done for them. These rocks served as concrete reminders of significant events, and they encouraged the retelling of stories of God's faithfulness. Today, we can use a pile of rocks as well, but we can also use other physical items. You might want to use objects of significance, such as an old photo album or journal, a worn-out baseball, a piece of jewelry, or any item that has personal meaning for the person.

Given the difficulty that those with Alzheimer's have with free recall (remembering without reminders), these physical objects should be placed prominently so the person with dementia can see them, and caregivers should use them to initiate discussion. Because memory failures can be a sensitive topic, avoid starting the conversation by saying, "Do you remember ..." Instead, use phrases that avoid "quizzing" the person. Start by saying something like, "Tell me about this picture" or "I remember the day when you ..." These phrases are less threatening and will encourage further conversation.

> God instructed the people to pile up the rocks as reminders to those who laid them and to future generations of what he had done for them. These rocks served as concrete reminders of significant events, and they encouraged the retelling of stories of God's faithfulness.

Comfort and connection in the moment is the goal of this kind of remembering, rather than seeking to develop new long-term memories. Caregivers and family members need to know that they are not doing this in the hope that it will be remembered tomorrow. This is a difficult shift to make. We must assume the person will forget this moment, and we will have to find ways to remind them anew each day. This leads us to consider the second method that God gives to help us remember.

The Role of Community in Remembering

God gives us other people—a community of believers—to remind us not only of who God is and what he has done, but also who we are in Christ. When a person develops significant cognitive impairment much of their life seems to revolve around their disease. It begins to redefine their identity and seems to be the truest thing about them. Yet this is not biblical. Scripture tells us that all who trust in Christ — including those with Alzheimer's — have a new identity. They are a new creation. They have value, regardless of their cognitive or intellectual ability. A spiritual community can remind us of this by treating us in ways that are consistent with this truth.

Those with dementia need guides to help them recall who they are. As we have seen, some long-term memories remain intact much longer than the more recent short-term memories. But in either case, prompting and cueing is still helpful. Remembering can be a social act. Our brothers and sisters play an important role in our collective remembering. We see this in the Old Testament when God taught his people how to remember his commands.

> These commandments that I give you today are to be on your hearts. Impress them on your children. Talk about them when you sit at home and when you walk along the road, when you lie down and when you get up. Tie them as symbols on your hands and bind them on your foreheads. Write them on the doorframes of your houses and on your gates. (Deuteronomy 6:6–9)

Though these verses directly speak of things parents should do with their children, they highlight the importance of remembering as a social act. Collectively, we are to work together to find ways of remembering, reminding each other and helping others to integrate the truths and presence of God into our lives. When remembrance is social, we remember much better than we do in isolation. As we remind each other we help each other maintain an outlook that is rooted in the faith we profess.

There are two key principles in this passage from Deuteronomy 6 that I want to highlight. Although these are also physical reminders, I want to point them out because they are best done in community with others.

Make a Routine of Remembering

When we make something a part of our daily routine we are less likely to forget it. People with dementia benefit from routines and rhythms in their daily life. This draws on procedural aspects of memory, which is largely spared in Alzheimer's. Reading Scripture, hymn singing, and prayer will have greater effect when they are incorporated into a daily routine.

Write It Down

God commanded the Israelites to write down his commandments and to put them in prominent places. They wrote them on their door-frames so they would see them as they left their homes and returned, and tied them on their foreheads so that Scripture would always be on their mind. God commanded them to write down the account of a critical battle and keep it on a scroll along with a jar of manna so they would be reminded of what the Lord had done in his faithfulness. In this case, a physical reminder (manna) is combined with a written account to aid in remembering.

If a person is in the middle or advanced stages of dementia, another person may need to write things down for them to help them remember in the moment. They may not remember you writing them down and might even be confused about the source of the writing, but you can explain this to them, even when they forget. You might help them write down parts of their story or you may write down key Bible verses, familiar prayers, or anything that might be familiar and comforting.

Again, the goal is not long-term memory development. It is remembering God moment to moment. These reminders prompt us to remember that God is faithful, never forgets his promises, and never fails to deliver.

Reading the Bible

The Bible is the authoritative source for God's story. Reading and listening to the Bible is the most basic spiritual discipline,[2] and, therefore, we incorporate it into the task of remembering. The words of Scripture are accessible and clear to us with the help of the Holy

Spirit.[3] Reading familiar passages and reminding people of God's story is a powerful way of helping people with Alzheimer's and their families remember the Lord. One pastor observed that familiar passages, particularly Psalms and stories from the life of Jesus, seem to be particularly powerful in ministering to people with severe memory impairment. They administer the Word of God and can spark older memories that encourage the person in their faith and bring a sense of peace.

One older man I knew had Alzheimer's as well as limited vision. He was a gentle and kind man who visited a dementia day center and was always happy to greet each person in the morning. His interaction was limited to answering questions about how he was doing and asking others the same. As the day wore on, he would get tired, and his poor vision and memory impairment would sometimes combine in an unhealthy blend, leading him to forget where he was. During these times he would become somewhat belligerent. He would yell and shake his cane at whoever walked by. He felt he was being held against his will, and since no one would take him home from this strange place, he felt the need to fight back. This was upsetting to the other people with dementia who saw him. As the staff considered how to address this problem, one remembered that he was a Christian and suggested that someone read the Bible with him. I remember his reaction clearly. I walked up next to him, acknowledged his situation, and asked if I could read the Bible to him while he waited for his ride home. He agreed. Though he was still not sure of who I was or what he was doing in this strange place, as I sat next to him and read the Bible, the anger melted away. Soon, he was nodding in agreement with the words of God, whispering, "That's right ... mmm hmm." When I finished, he still didn't know where he was or who I was, but he thanked me. For him, God's Word was an anchor in the storm of his confusion. Reminded of the Lord's goodness, he experienced peace.

Remembering through Music

Church services incorporate music into their liturgy to help engage us in the collective remembrance of the gospel story.[4] Memory for music and songs is surprisingly resilient, even in advanced Alzheimer's. Churches and families can take advantage of these relatively spared procedural and emotional memory systems, which include memory for familiar music and lyrics. People with dementia can often recall lines and melodies from songs long into the course of the disease. It is not uncommon to see a person with advanced dementia deeply moved by an old hymn, even if that person's (declarative) memory impairment will lead them to forget it all just moments later. Again, the comfort and connection in the moment is, in itself, a valuable goal. The fact that it may soon be forgotten should not diminish its value.

I remember the first time I saw someone with Alzheimer's remembering the Lord through music. I was working in a day center that provided meaningful activities for people with dementia. The full range of dementia was represented, from those who rarely spoke and stared straight ahead to mildly impaired people who were able to help take care of others. Some could not speak comprehensible words and had trouble understanding what others told them. Some were joyful and content, while others were anxious and agitated, wanting to go home, even if they didn't know where that was anymore.

When it came time for music, and especially the old hymns, things visibly changed. One woman who only wanted to leave finally sat down for a while to listen. A man who was always angry and agitated now had a contented look and tapped his foot to the music. Another man who was quite confused closed his tear-filled eyes and slowly raised his hands while quietly mouthing each word. God uses music to reach the seemingly unreachable. And he gives us this gift as a gracious resource to help us in drawing people back to him, to reengage in their faith.

Communion

In 1 Corinthians 11, Paul tells us that remembering is one of the reasons we celebrate the Lord's Supper, or Communion:

> For I received from the Lord what I also passed on to you: The Lord Jesus, on the night he was betrayed, took bread, and when he had

given thanks, he broke it and said, "This is my body, which is for you; do this in remembrance of me." In the same way, after supper he took the cup, saying, "This cup is the new covenant in my blood; do this, whenever you drink it, in remembrance of me." For whenever you eat this bread and drink this cup, you proclaim the Lord's death until he comes. (vv. 23–26)

Communion is a present act that reminds us of what Christ did for us in the past and what he promises for us in the future. Whatever difficulties we currently face, this simple reminder helps us to see the present as part of a larger reality. One pastor pointed out how Communion can help us remember God's faithfulness in the midst of deep difficulty and a desire to be healed:

> *When we are overwhelmed by a sense of our sinfulness, or our prayers for healing seem to bounce back off the ceiling, or we're stuck at the bottom of the pit, or we are crowned with despair and desolation, or when one bad thing after another batters our lives and flying on eagles' wings is an impossible dream, it is easy to forget all his benefits. In this simple but powerful picture, the Lord's Supper calls us back to the center of it all and to the vast benefits that flow to us from the cross of Christ.*[5]

As a sacrament, Communion can be shared with Christians who have Alzheimer's to give them a concrete reminder of Christ and his sacrifice for us. Communion should be taken in an appropriate fashion, with those administering it reminding those who partake of the purpose of the sacrament and how it will proceed (as is done in many church services). Those administering it may also encourage the person to "examine oneself" (see 1 Corinthians 11:28) by reminding the person of Christ's sacrifice for sins and by encouraging them to take a moment to confess their sin to the Lord either together in a general prayer of confession, led by the person administering, or silently.

Even though people may forget explicit information and be unable to explain what Communion means, there is a good possibility that they implicitly remember how to take Communion since the procedural and emotional memory systems may be spared. Again, the benefit is in the moment. Those receiving Communion will likely have some recollection of what it means and why they are doing it, even if they cannot communicate this after the fact.[6]

Both music and Communion rely on multiple sensory inputs: hearing, vision, touch, and even taste. It may seem obvious that using multiple avenues to reach people with brain impairment is a good idea, but sometimes we overlook the obvious. Whatever efforts you make in prompting memories of the Lord, don't forget that you are dealing with people who have memory systems that are heavily damaged. No single key exists to unlock the past. These efforts will work unevenly at best—sometimes the person will seem to connect with one way but not another, and sometimes what worked one week will not work the next. Keep trying multiple routes into the person's memory. Smells, tastes, sounds, and pictures may prompt memory in ways that words do not.[7]

Prayer

One chaplain described a woman in the middle stages of dementia who would exclaim, "Thank God you're here. I love the Lord!" whenever she walked into the memory-care unit. As her dementia progressed, her ability to communicate declined, and she could no longer speak in a way that was understandable. Instead, she would scream and yell, which was disturbing to other residents. But the chaplain knew she was a faithful Catholic, and one day he decided to bring her a rosary. The screaming woman gently took it and began to pray, clearly and just loud enough to hear. The screaming was gone, replaced by well-known prayers of faith. From that point on, whenever the screaming would resume, the staff of the unit would bring her rosary to her, and in prayer she would find peace.

Some Cautions

Although these methods are evidences of God's grace in helping us remember, and we should expect God to do great things, a word of caution is in order. Sometimes we hear about a new way of interacting or treating a person with dementia, and we think it is the magic pill that will fix things. You might do some of the things I've mentioned here only to find that the person does not respond, at least not in any way you can see. Or one method will seem to spark remembrance one day but not another. Some prompt remembrance while others receive no response. One caregiver illustrated this reality to me:

> During my last visit, Mother and I attended church at the facility where she lives. The pastor was passing the Communion elements and when he got to my mother, she had no idea what to do with the small cup of juice or cube of bread. How many times in her life had she taken Communion? Countless. And now she did not know what to do! The reality of that made me cry, right then and there. Graciously the pastor placed the bread in her mouth and assisted her with the cup. As the service went on, she looked like she was sleeping. We got to the hymn after the sermon, and do you know she sang every word of all the verses with her eyes shut? It was as if God were saying, "What you can see with your eyes is not the way it is!" She looked asleep and seemed out of touch, and yet she sang every word of praise to her God. God didn't need to provide that for me, but he did. Does that change my thoughts about her spiritual connection and ability to remember? Absolutely.

God pursues us in love, and we are called to do the same with people with dementia, helping to engage them in remembering the Lord. These are not techniques for drilling facts and reminders into a person's head. These are spiritual practices that we should seek to integrate into the rhythms of daily life.

Seek the Guidance of the Spirit

We have already mentioned the role of the Holy Spirit as a helper and how we work in concert with the Spirit to help people remember. We should pray for the Holy Spirit to move in the hearts and minds of people with dementia, trusting that God may have provision for them that we have not considered. The Lord is at work in believers

Prayers for Those with Alzheimer's

Here are some suggestions offered by families for how to pray for someone with Alzheimer's disease:

Pray that the Lord will calm the confusion

Pray for relief from anxiety and for peace

Pray that the Lord will strengthen the person for what the Lord has for them that day

Pray that they will experience the Lord as their shepherd

Pray for comfort through the day and night

Pray for assurance that the person is a child of the King and that nothing can take that away

Pray that the Lord will be with us and carry the person's inner burdens

Pray for relief from pain and loneliness

Pray for a peaceful transition from this earthly home to the heavenly home (for those nearing death)

with dementia, helping them to remember who he is, even when we, as those who love and care for people with dementia, do not see it.

Until Jesus returns, the Holy Spirit plays a critical role in "bearing witness to Christ-followers that they truly belong to God forever (Romans 8:16)."[8] This is a true comfort in the depths of Alzheimer's disease — which so often seems to reach into the very core of our being — that the Holy Spirit, who is not only unseen but eternal, can offer us comfort, hope, and remembrance of the goodness of the gospel and our true hope in grace. By the Spirit "we cry, '*Abba*, Father.' The Spirit himself testifies with our spirit that we are God's children" (Romans 8:15 – 16).

We should commit to pray that the Holy Spirit will cause people with Alzheimer's to remember the Lord and what he has done for

Prayers for Caregivers

Here are some ways to pray for those who give care to those with Alzheimer's:

Pray for patience and strength

Pray for knowledge, understanding, and insights about how to provide the best care

Pray for peace and the ability to accept their role as a caregiver

Pray for times of rest and respite, including time to be alone with God

Pray for help and support from others — family, friends, church

Pray for wisdom in decision making and the ability to prioritize

Pray for humility and the willingness to ask for help when it is needed

Pray for the Lord to provide specific verses or passages of Scripture that will encourage

Pray for flexibility as the care needs seem to change, sometimes moment to moment

Pray for the Lord to provide prayer partners and friendships

them. The person may not be able to verbalize these memories, but we might encounter them in moments of peace, in the brief smile of contentment, or even a gentle touch. Knowing God gives peace that surpasses all understanding to those of us on the outside looking in. The memory might be quickly forgotten, but this does not invalidate that momentary remembrance.

We should pray that the Lord will help them remember who they are because they are in Christ — the old has gone and the new has come (2 Corinthians 5:17). Though the brain may be fading away, this new self and new creation is being formed in the likeness of Christ through the Holy Spirit in preparation for full restoration.

Christ provides the comfort that our hearts long for through the presence of the Holy Spirit. As we offer our presence and comfort to those with Alzheimer's, we must remind ourselves that the Holy Spirit has gone before us and is already at work. God's work begins long before ours does.

Initiate and Invite

A pastor recalled meeting with a ninety-year-old woman with dementia who seemed so impaired that her family doubted he would be able to communicate with her. His plan was simple. He shared some well-known Scripture verses with her (Psalm 23 and 121, and John 3:16) and then began to play the old, well-known hymn "The Old Rugged Cross." The woman's memory for the Lord was on grand display, as she soon joined in singing each word with this pastor. As the pastor said to me, "As her daughter looked on, she was totally captivated and mesmerized that her mother could remember."

As fellow believers drawn into community with people who have Alzheimer's, we are called to help them remember. When a person has dementia they may not initiate faith practices or conversations. The role of the church is to help point the person (and their family) to God's sovereignty and work, emphasizing that grace is never about what we do, but what God has

> The role of the church is to help point the person (and their family) to God's sovereignty and work, emphasizing that grace is never about what we do, but what God has already done. Even though they may not be able to do what they once did, faith is always about God's grace.

already done. Even though they may not be able to do what they once did, faith is always about God's grace.

We play a role in inviting them into the exercise of the faith that they hold and have held for years. If you are caring for a loved one who has not believed in the past, your task is a bit different, but it should follow the same pattern. You can invite them into a journey of faith while providing loving, grace-filled care, and praying that the Lord will move in their heart. It is the Holy Spirit who must move first. We cannot and should not pressure anyone to believe. But remember, your loving care, motivated by the grace of Christ and guided by the Holy Spirit, is a powerful witness.

> Even when Alzheimer's seems to strip away so much from our lives, we still find that God is there. He never changes, he is always present, and he never forgets.

God initiates and we respond. You can begin to see how this might work for people with dementia. When you initiate faith practices, those who have believed often respond quite movingly. This is a demonstration of how God can work in them and through us. How much more will they respond quietly to the working of the Spirit, which we cannot see?

In Alzheimer's we see clearly that although we are limited, God provides what we need. It isn't about us and what we can do — it never was. It is about what God has done through his Son, Jesus, and how he continues to sustain us through the unseen working of the Holy Spirit. Even when Alzheimer's seems to strip away so much from our lives, we still find that God is there. He never changes, he is always present, and he never forgets.

• •
FOR FURTHER REFLECTION

Chapter 3 taught us about the different types of memory and the current chapter builds on this by explaining how we can help people with Alzheimer's disease remember the Lord. Think about the last church service you attended.

- Which aspects of the service do you think would be most effective in reaching a person with Alzheimer's disease? Which parts would be most difficult? What about the physical environment — do you think it helps or hinders the person with dementia?

- If you were going to design a church service for people with Alzheimer's and their families, what would it look like?

- How can you bring the church to people who have Alzheimer's and no longer attend services?

- What does the forgetting observed in Alzheimer's disease teach us about God's grace?

• •

Chapter 10

PREVENTION AND PLANNING

Many people who learn about Alzheimer's disease or experience its devastating effects in the life of a loved one wonder what they can do to prevent its onset in the first place. Many in their middle and later years live in the shadow of fear that they will develop some form of dementia. They take up crossword puzzles or play Sudoku in hopes that it will stave off the devastating effects. Assuming you do not currently have Alzheimer's or a form of cognitive loss, is there anything you can do to prevent it?

In this chapter, we'll take a two-pronged approach to help those without Alzheimer's think about various ways of taking action to prevent the disease and look at the science related to prevention. We will also discuss things you can do to prepare for Alzheimer's disease, that is, ways of planning for the future. How would you want to live if you were someday to develop this condition? How do you want to live now in light of this possibility in the future?

Much has been written about "ending well." But let's think about what it would mean to "end well" if our ending involves Alzheimer's. This disease strips away so much from us, and forces us to evaluate what is most important. As we move into our later years, we are reminded that it is good to plan, but it is ultimately the Lord who determines our steps (Proverbs 16:1–4). There is nothing wrong with planning, but we must never forget that it is the Lord who is in control. As we discuss planning, we must submit our plans to him, making them in faith — not in fear.

> Many in their middle and later years live in the shadow of fear that they will develop some form of dementia.... Assuming you do not currently have Alzheimer's or a form of cognitive loss, is there anything you can do to prevent it?

Can It Be Prevented?

Preventing Alzheimer's disease is a complicated endeavor. New research emerges almost every week, suggesting that we should eat more berries, drink a special kind of tea, or play certain computer games — all of which are said to hold off dementia. How are we to make sense of this? Who should we listen to? Before you get blueberry stains on your video-game controller, consider the current scientific evidence.

Hundreds of research studies have examined risk factors for and prevention of Alzheimer's disease and other cognitive disorders. Since the quality of this research varies widely, we'll focus our attention on research that has been the most carefully reviewed.[1]

Let's begin by looking at some of the factors that can increase risk for developing Alzheimer's. Some risk factors are fixed — we cannot change our genes, for example — while others can be changed, such as our diet or level of activity. The most consistent and powerful risk factor is one that none of us can control: advancing age. As people live longer they increase their chances of getting Alzheimer's or other dementias. Growing older increases the risk far more than any of the modifiable risk factors. In fact, the rate of Alzheimer's and dementia doubles every five years you age beyond sixty-five.

A consensus report from a panel of experts summarized some of the most consistent findings in the research.[2] They found that smoking, depression, diabetes, metabolic syndrome[3] and the *apolipoprotein e4* (APOE e4) gene were associated with increased risk for cognitive decline. Although genetics is a risk factor, it is not as strong as most people suspect. If you have a first-degree relative—parent, sibling, or child—with Alzheimer's, your risk is two to four times greater than a person without a first-degree relative with Alzheimer's. This also changes depending on age and other factors. Still, it appears that Alzheimer's is not determined solely by genes. Except in the case of early-onset Alzheimer's disease (onset before age sixty-five), which is rarer than late-onset (around 250 thousand of the 5 million Americans with Alzheimer's), most of the genes related to the disease are what we would call *susceptibility* genes. These are genetic markers (like the widely researched APOE gene) that increase susceptibility for the condition but do not determine whether you will get it. Because of this, it is not typically recommended that you seek out genetic testing for this gene.[4] Many have noted that the mere presence of a gene is no guarantee that you will develop Alzheimer's disease.[5]

There are also some promising findings related to prevention. Cognitive training and engagement, vegetable intake, high levels of physical activity, engagement in leisure activity, higher omega-3 fatty acid intake, and a Mediterranean diet have all been associated with lower risk of cognitive decline. Taken together, this suggests that there are several steps you can take to help reduce your risk for Alzheimer's disease, although doing these things will not *eliminate* your risk altogether. All of these also have beneficial effects on health and well-being in other ways. This means that if you do them, they will help you, even if someday the scientific literature goes the other direction and finds they do not, in fact, lower Alzheimer's risk. In other words, you have nothing to lose!

To help prevent Alzheimer's consider the following:

- If you smoke, stop now. If you don't smoke, don't start.
- Eat a healthy diet with low saturated fat and low in sugar and with lots of vegetables.
- Remain cognitively engaged as you age.
- Engage in high levels of physical activity.
- Adjust your lifestyle to help you avoid diabetes, high blood pressure, and high cholesterol.
- If you already have these conditions, don't ignore them. Take active steps to manage them well under the direction of a physician.

The research does not suggest that we can fully prevent cognitive decline and dementia. But we can be good stewards of the bodies and brains God has given us, and in doing so, we can reduce some of the risk of cognitive decline, perhaps lessening the amount of cognitive and functional changes experienced and maybe delaying their onset. Keep that in mind as you make choices about what you eat and drink and how you take care of your body and brain. By the time you reach your later years, you'll be living with the physiological effects of the choices you have made over the past sixty to seventy years, and these effects can accumulate over time and impact the health and resiliency of your brain.

You can take other steps that may have some *limited* benefit in reducing risk for cognitive decline. The absence of social support, for example, has been associated with greater risk of Alzheimer's. *Social support* is the scientific term for having people around you who love and care for you when you need it. This might be many people or a few close confidants — people you can go to when you need someone to talk to, share your pain, fears, or other trials with, or even just go to when you need help. People who report that they have this are generally physically healthier, have a better sense of well-being, and are more resistant to the negative effects of stress. It now appears that they may also have a lower risk of Alzheimer's. Furthermore, emerging research suggests that people who are lonely have double the risk of Alzheimer's disease.[6] In other words, it is not good to be alone (Genesis 2:18).

So what about doing crossword puzzles, Sudoku, and the plethora of video games claiming to hold off cognitive decline? Although there is growing evidence that these can be helpful,[7] these may simply be another form of cognitive activity and engagement, as cited above. These fall in a wide range of activities that can help to keep you engaged and active. If you enjoy them and can afford them, they may be helpful. But many people begrudgingly do these activities daily without enjoyment because they are hoping to hold off dementia. I understand the sentiment behind this, but in truth these activities are unlikely to be that effective over the long haul. If you have options for engaging in activities, ask yourself if this is how you want to spend your days. Is there more to life than holding off decline? Is this living life to the fullest? Since our days are numbered, we should think carefully about how to live them.

Preparing for Alzheimer's

Many people spend time and effort and, sometimes, considerable amounts of money on prevention, but they neglect to plan. If you worry about developing dementia down the road, take some time to think about how you might prepare for it. If you have some genetic risk for Alzheimer's, know that even if your parent had it you still have a better chance of *not* getting it than you do of getting it. With that in mind, know that you do have a greater risk than others, so it doesn't hurt to take time to help yourself and your family by prayerfully developing a plan. Recent estimates suggest that one in three older people die with Alzheimer's.[8] I believe it would be wise for all of us to plan ahead, even if we never end up developing the disease.

Several areas are typically considered when planning for Alzheimer's disease. These include legal and financial matters, care preferences, and end-of-life issues. At minimum, everyone should have an *advanced directive*, either in the form of a living will, specifying what type of medical care is wanted or unwanted at the end of life, and the designation of durable power of attorney, designating who will make decisions for you in the event that you become unable to. Be sure to plan for what will happen with your money and property. This can be done through a will or living trust.

After a person develops dementia their capacity to make decisions becomes questionable, so thinking about these things now and talking with your family about them will help avoid problems in the future. It might be helpful to document these decisions with the aid of an elder-law specialist. From a medical perspective, this is also the time to think about and discuss with your family what you want in terms of medical care if you were to develop advanced dementia. Often these discussions are focused on what level of care you would want to receive, including more aggressive attempts to keep you alive, such as respirators, feeding tubes, CPR, IV hydration, and antibiotics.[9]

Planning for Living

There is more to planning than deciding who will get your money, what treatments you would want, and who will make decisions for you when you can't. Preparing for Alzheimer's also should include asking how you want to live in light of everything we've discussed up to this point.

If you learned today that you would develop Alzheimer's in five, ten, or even twenty years, how would you want to live your life until that time and then after you were diagnosed? In Psalm 90:12, Moses writes, "Teach us to number our days, that we may gain a heart of wisdom." There is wisdom to this, knowing that our days are already numbered. It forces us to consider more carefully how we might live in our remaining days. Again, we should recognize that not everyone develops Alzheimer's, but what if you did?

Some research has focused on how people perceive the time they have left and how this affects their thinking and emotions. When we perceive that we have less time left to live, we tend to shift our focus away from achievement-oriented goals and focus on social and emotional goals.[10] In a sense, ambitious strivings tend to decline and people decide they want spend more time on what is really important to them, including the people they love. Thinking about time makes a difference in how we prioritize and evaluate our lives.

What would you do if you had just a year to live? What would you do with your time if you won the lottery and no longer needed to work? These "what if" types of questions are common and have a way of refocusing our thoughts on what is important and lasting. They encourage us to imagine and reevaluate our priorities and beliefs concerning life and its meaning. In light of what you've learned about Alzheimer's disease, ask yourself:

- How would I want to live if I were diagnosed with Alzheimer's disease?
- How would I want to live right now if I knew I was going to develop Alzheimer's disease?
- How would I want people to care for me if I knew I couldn't care for myself?
- How would I want people to treat me if I couldn't remember?
- Who would I want to be with?
- How would I want to spend my time?
- Where would I want to be?
- What would I want to be sure that I always remembered?

These questions reflect some of the broader life questions we mentioned:

- What is really important to me?
- Who is really important to me?
- What do I want to remember?
- Who do I want to remember?
- If I could distill my life down to a few elements that I never wanted to forget, what would they be?
- What matters most in life?

This is the time to discuss the practical aspects of living and dying with Alzheimer's, but it is also the time to reconsider what is most important to you. No one knows exactly what it will be like to experience dementia personally until it actually happens. Take time to consider, pray over, and discuss these things with your family and friends. It will benefit you and them in the long run. You may even find that considering these things changes your perspective on how you want to live today, bringing you closer to God and to those he has placed around you.

In considering what is important in life, recall the words of Jesus as he summarized the law, which guides us in how to live:

> "Teacher, which is the greatest commandment in the Law?"
>
> Jesus replied: " 'Love the Lord your God with all your heart and with all your soul and with all your mind.' This is the first and greatest commandment. And the second is like it: 'Love your neighbor as yourself.' All the Law and the Prophets hang on these two commandments." (Matthew 22:36–40)

What does it look like to love God and love others when you live with Alzheimer's disease? Looking forward, how can you plan to live this way? How do you want to love and walk with God while you are older? If you were to develop memory problems, how would you continue doing this? Who can you love and who will help you continue in your faith walk?

When you think about how you would like to live, walking each day with the Lord and others as you grow older, think about what this might look like and make a plan for implementing this now, for you will surely not make and implement these things once you develop Alzheimer's disease or become a caregiver. Aging well does not begin when you turn sixty-five—it is a lifelong process, and it is best to start early.

> Aging well does not begin when you turn sixty-five — it is a lifelong process, and it is best to start early.

Planning to Remember

Are there certain passages of Scripture or songs that lift your heart and give you hope in difficult times? What passages are embedded in your heart? What are the parts of your story that you would want to remember?

When people prepare for the possibility of Alzheimer's they often operate under the assumption that remembering will not be possible. As we have seen, there are ways to remember. It is wise to prepare since God helps us remember and frequently calls us to do so.

Remember the Lord's faithfulness and how he has called you to live. Remember your story, rehearse it, and review how God has worked and been faithful in your life. He has worked and been present in past trials, and he will do so again in the future. Reviewing, remembering, and consolidating now will provide comfort in the future.

Plan for Community

Do you want to be embedded in a loving church who will care for you when you can no longer care for yourself? Do you want to be surrounded by people who share the same faith and hope that you profess?

We often lack a deep understanding of one another in today's fast-paced world. If you fear developing Alzheimer's disease, take some time to develop a deeper understanding of those you love and let them understand you as well. Sometimes it seems that it takes something big and tragic to force us to let down our guard and be truly vulnerable with one another. But Alzheimer's can develop so slowly and gradually that by the time people realize that they are facing it, it may be too late to really have this type of meeting of the hearts. (It isn't that they can't; it's just much more difficult.) Take advantage of the present to be open and vulnerable. Remember together—let your testimony encourage one another.

Consider now whether you can make peace in any broken relationships. If you have relationship conflict, whether old hurts or unaddressed issues, seek God's guidance in addressing them now, because this will become increasingly difficult to do down the road, particularly if you develop dementia. When these relationship issues are carried forward into dementia, it makes it more difficult for people to take care of each other and there is some research to suggest that caregivers in these situations experience a much greater burden.[11] Resolving old conflicts is difficult and tricky, and we must pray for God's grace to heal these and for the Holy Spirit to guide us.

> If it is possible, as far as it depends on you, live at peace with everyone. (Romans 12:18)

The letter to the Hebrews encourages us to "make every effort to live in peace with everyone" (12:14). This recognizes that even our best efforts to make peace may not always work out. Resolving conflicts and making peace becomes even more difficult — though not impossible — when dementia develops.

Develop Godly Habits

We are saved by grace. We cannot save ourselves by behaving well. Yet God still calls us to holiness for our own good. In following him, our character and faith walk are further developed, and this will serve us well as we age. We can either make a habit of things that are good for us or of things that are not good for us, but either way, these repeated patterns of behavior become deeply embedded. Scholar and author N. T. Wright develops this in his book on Christian character and virtue:

> *Virtue ... is what happens when someone has made a thousand small choices, requiring effort and concentration, to do something which is good and right but which doesn't "come naturally" — and then, on the thousand and first time, when it really matters, they find that they do what's required "automatically," as we say. On that thousand and first occasion, it does indeed look as if it "just happens"; but reflection tells us that it doesn't "just happen" as easily as that.... Virtue is what happens when wise and courageous choices have become "second nature."*[12]

What aspects of your walk with God would you want to become "second nature"? Which memories and actions would you want to be so reflexive that you would be more likely to continue to do them — even when you have cognitive problems? People with Alzheimer's disease live out habits each day, just as people without Alzheimer's do. There is evidence, in fact, that some behavioral problems in dementia are linked with past personality and character traits.[13] Families often report that the behavioral issues they face with a loved one with dementia are intensifications of traits the person had before dementia. Similarly, relationship conflicts in dementia are sometimes an intensification or continuation of prior relationship conflicts.

> We are being formed by what we do today. The things that we do not only can affect our risk for dementia but also influence who we become in terms of our character and our habits.

By choosing how to live now, we are making choices about how we will live in the future. We are being formed by the things that we do. Who do you want to be? Who do you want to share your future years of life with? How can you make peace with others? How will you have the mind of Christ, with the Word planted deep in your heart so that it will always be upon your lips? Do you have a habit of daily prayer and Scripture reading? In developing godly habits we make them a part of who we are and embed them in our souls and procedural memory systems. All of these are more resistant to the effects of Alzheimer's disease.

Consistently making the spiritual disciplines a part of your daily walk will be beneficial in growing in your knowledge of God and your understanding of his Word.[14] Remembering his goodness will not only benefit you, but also those you share these memories with. These are good things regardless of whether you develop Alzheimer's. If you do, these things may remain with you, and those you have loved can remind you of these things when you forget.

Consider the following resolutions made by Pastor John Piper as he spent time considering what it means to age with God in light of the words of Psalm 71 (NRSV). If you are living with the possibility of Alzheimer's disease, these same resolutions are worthy of consideration and meditation. How can you creatively and systematically integrate these into your daily life so that they can come naturally once your memory begins to fail?

1. I will remember with wonder and thanks the thousands of times I have leaned on God since my youth. "For you, O LORD, are my hope, my trust, O LORD, from my youth. Upon you I have leaned from my birth" (verses 5–6). "O God from my youth you have taught me, and I still proclaim your wondrous deeds" (verse 17).

2. I will take refuge in God rather than taking offense at my troubles. "In you, O LORD, I take refuge" (verse 1).

3. I will speak to God more and more (not less and less) of all his greatness until there is no room in my mouth for murmuring. "My praise is continually of you" (verse 6). "I will praise you yet more and more" (verse 14).

4. I will hope (doggedly) and not give in to despair, even in the nursing home, and even if I outlive all my friends. "I will hope continually" (verse 14).

5. I will find people to tell about God's wonderful acts of salvation, and never run out, because they are innumerable. "My mouth will tell of your righteous acts, of your deeds of salvation all day long, though their number is past my knowledge" (verse 15). "I proclaim your might to all the generations to come" (verse 18).

6. I will remember that there are great things about God above my imagination, and soon enough I will know these too. "Your power and your righteousness, O God, reach the high heavens" (verse 18).

7. I will count all my pain and troubles as a gift from God and a path to glory. "You who have made me see many troubles and calamities will revive me again" (verse 20).

8. I will resist stereotypes of old people, and play and sing and shout with joy (whether I look dignified or not). "I will also praise you with the harp for your faithfulness, O my God; I will sing praises to you with the lyre, O Holy One of Israel" (verse 22). "My lips will shout for joy, when I sing praises to you" (verse 23).[15]

Prayerfully consider how you can write your own care manual in which you can lay out what is important and how you'd like to live. Pray for God to guide you in this. Let your plan be sacrificial, thinking of others before yourself. You don't want to develop a plan that those who might care for you could never accomplish. Discuss this with them, pray over it, and plan together. Then take action.

We are being formed by what we do today. The things that we do not only can affect our risk for dementia but also influence who we become in terms of our character and our habits. We have little control over whether we will develop dementia, but we can influence our level of risk. Planning for the future also involves what you want to do and who you want to be. We need to think about how our character and faith are developed so that when trouble comes, we are rooted deeply in Christ and surrounded by his Holy Spirit.

FOR FURTHER REFLECTION

In this chapter we learned about how we are being formed by what we choose to do today, both in terms of our character and our risk for dementia.

- What can you change about your current life that might reduce your risk for dementia? How can you become a better steward of your brain?

- Knowing that Alzheimer's disease cannot be fully prevented, take steps toward planning by answering the following questions and share your answers with someone you love:

- How would I want to live if I were diagnosed with Alzheimer's disease?

- How would I want people to care for me if I knew I couldn't care for myself?

- How would I want to live right now if I knew I was going to develop Alzheimer's disease?

- What would I want to be sure that I always remembered?

Chapter 11

GOD NEVER FORGETS

Lewis had gotten so bad that even those who knew him best could no longer tell what he remembered. He rarely spoke, and when he did, it was often a grunt or groan. He could barely walk and relied upon his wife to wheel him from room to room. He had grown too heavy to support his own weight. Swallowing became difficult, and he often choked on his food, breaking into full-body spasms that terrified both of them.

In the early years of their Alzheimer's journey, Lewis and his wife had prayed every day for healing, in hopes that God would work a miracle. By now, Lewis had stopped speaking audible prayers, and though Ann was holding on to hope and faith, there were times where she couldn't fight off the feeling that they had been forgotten.

How long, LORD? Will you forget me forever?
How long will you hide your face from me?
How long must I wrestle with my thoughts
and day after day have sorrow in my heart?

How long will my enemy triumph over me?
Look on me and answer, LORD my God.
  Give light to my eyes, or I will sleep in death,
and my enemy will say, "I have overcome him,"
  and my foes will rejoice when I fall. (Psalm 13:1–4)

It can seem as if Alzheimer's and other dementias defeat us in the end. They are an enemy that progressively steals from our lives until we die, confused and alone, ending our years with a moan (Psalm 90:9). To combat these fears and doubts, we have only the promises of God to cling to.

But I trust in your unfailing love;
  my heart rejoices in your salvation.
I will sing the LORD's praise,
  for he has been good to me. (Psalm 13:5–6)

Though it may seem as if the Lord has forgotten us, we cling to the underlying truth that although we forget our Creator and Redeemer, he never forgets us. He always remembers us, fully knows us, and sustains us, even as we approach the end of this earthly life. Even as we fall into a state of seemingly hopeless decay, we know that God remembers his children and mercifully calls us home.

God Doesn't Forget

We've discussed the importance of remembering the Lord, how he has been at work throughout redemptive history and in our individual lives. When we remember him, we find a place to anchor our lives as we are battered about by the suffering of dementia.

But we also find comfort in knowing that even in our forgetting, God doesn't forget.[1] He continues to know us. In fact,

> But we also find comfort in knowing that even in our forgetting, God doesn't forget.... In fact, it is far more significant that God remembers us than that we remember him.

it is far more significant that God remembers us than that we remember him. This speaks to the reality that our salvation, from beginning to end, is by grace. In grace God reaches out to rescue us—not the other way around. Our salvation, ultimately, is not up to us. We cannot save ourselves. And there is comfort in this as a person experiences physical and mental decay. We continue to have hope that they are moving closer to full restoration. It is not necessary for them to be able to articulate this hope

> God remembers and knows us more deeply than we could ever imagine — we are never out of his mind. Even when others forget us, God does not.

for it to be true. God loves them just as much now as when they were born and when they first believed. God's love covers our sin and our forgetting with full knowledge of all that we have done and will do. There is no discovery or development that can diminish God's view of us, even the devastation that Alzheimer's wreaks upon our brains. As Van Voorst writes,

> As rich as these usages of human remembering are, they are overshadowed by the richness of the more dominant Old Testament witness to the fact that God remembers. A scan through a Hebrew concordance or an analytical English concordance's listings for "remember" shows that the vast majority refer to God's remembering, not ours.[2]

God remembers and knows us more deeply than we could ever imagine—we are never out of his mind. Even when others forget us, God does not. One chaplain shared that she takes comfort in God's steadfastness and his promise to "never leave or forsake" us (see Deuteronomy 31:6; Joshua 1:5; Hebrews 13:5) as well as the words from Isaiah 49:16, "See, I have engraved you on the palms of my hands." She notes that people with Alzheimer's and other dementias are sometimes forgotten by their church and family. But God remains steadfast, never forgetting even one of his people, even when they are hidden away in a memory unit of a nursing home. Though they are locked away from the view of the world, God sees them.

Going Home

Visit an Alzheimer's day center or memory-care unit and you will inevitably hear the questions and pleas:

"When am I going home?"

"I want to go home."

"I need to get home."

These are repeated in various ways throughout the day, and they seem to gradually increase in frequency and intensity as the day drags on. This may be a longing for a literal physical structure that they once called home, but it is also a longing for a place that is familiar, comfortable, and secure—where they feel like they belong and are loved deeply and unconditionally.

We all share in this longing. As life drags on and our suffering increases, this plea to return home grows stronger. Those who belong to Christ may recall his promise to prepare a place for us. We long to be with our Creator, the source of all that is beautiful and lovely. We long to leave the pain of this life and to be with him.

When people with dementia ask for their home, they are expressing this deep longing for a place of belonging, acceptance, and security. Psalm 90 tells us, along with 2 Corinthians, that our home is in the Lord.

Lord, you have been our dwelling place throughout all generations. (Psalm 90:1)

Therefore we are always confident and know that as long as we are at home in the body we are away from the Lord. For we live by faith, not by sight. We are confident, I say, and would prefer to be away from the body and at home with the Lord. (2 Corinthians 5:6–8)

This longing for home is in our hearts, and we feel it over the years, decades, and generations. In a sense, we have known this longing for home ever since the fall, when Adam and Eve left the garden where they had walked with God in the coolness of the day. Sin led to our exile, and we were forced to leave the security of our home, the place where we belonged. Instead of joining God on a walk, human beings now hide from him in shame. But Christ has opened the door to us again, and one day he will return to take us home to his presence. As St. Augustine wrote, "You have made us for yourself, O Lord, and our heart is restless until it rests in you."[3]

Only in the Lord do we find true rest, the place of security and belonging. Until that day, we long and groan for the promised restoration not only for the healing of our bodies and brains but to experience the Lord fully—to see him and know him better, and once again walk with him in the cool of the day. What will that home look like?

> And I heard a loud voice from the throne saying, "Look! God's dwelling place is now among the people, and he will dwell with them. They will be his people, and God himself will be with them and be their God. 'He will wipe every tear from their eyes. There will be no more death' or mourning or crying or pain, for the old order of things has passed away."
>
> He who was seated on the throne said, "I am making everything new!" (Revelation 21:3–5)

One day we will be home again, dwelling with the Lord—the ultimate fulfillment of all of his promises. There will be no more death, mourning, crying, or pain. There will be no more agitation, no more wandering and getting lost, no more resisting care, no more confusion, no more delusions, no more screaming, and no more fears for what the future holds. Apathy will be replaced with rejoicing and anxiety with perfect peace.

And there will be no more forgetting. In fact, we will not need to remember the Lord and his goodness and promises, because we will experience these as we rejoice in his presence.

I met a man named John while I was writing this book, not knowing that within several months he would die. When we first met, he and his wife

In his prayer for me John said, "Help him to cling to you when he has nothing else to cling to." It was a fitting prayer from a person who seemed to have had everything stripped away by dementia.

shared their faith and glimpses of their story with me. Despite a decade of progressive loss, they testified to the goodness of God, his faithfulness, and their deep conviction that he had a plan. We prayed together, I for them, and they for me. In his prayer for me John said, "Help him to cling to you when he has nothing else to cling to." It was a fitting prayer from a person who seemed to have had everything stripped away by dementia.

Before I left him, John wanted to share a dream he had a few weeks earlier. At that time, John could hardly walk or take care of any of the basic activities of daily living due to his disease. In his dream, he found that his feet were beginning to wiggle. Soon after his feet started wiggling, he heard music in the distance. He arose and walked three flights of stairs to investigate. As he neared the end of the stairway, he heard the music much more clearly, and he saw walkways of shimmering gold. There were people rejoicing and dancing and having what John called a "real boogie party." His wife interjected at that point that John was once quite a dancer. "I could do it all" he told me with a proud smile.

Just a few months after he shared this dream with me, John's eyes glazed over and his heart rate dropped. He didn't eat or drink for the next two days, and he was confined to a hospital bed they had purchased for their home. Though he was able to converse, his face was expressionless. His wife knew the end was near.

John cried out to the Lord to give him "a little more time." Later that same day he was able to talk on the phone with one of his children, and he was at peace. The day after that, two friends traveled to see him, pray with him, and listen carefully to his remaining words of wisdom while they fed him ice cream spoonful by spoonful.

When the dementia had first taken hold of him, over a decade earlier, John had experienced dramatic mood swings and would often became enraged. No one could seem to reason with him. It had been a long, painful road, one that was physically and emotionally exhausting. Now, in his final days, his words were filled with gentleness, love, and grace. Just before he passed away, John turned to his wife and in a final gift of grace told her, "When I'm gone, you're going to be relieved. Don't feel guilty about it. You've done a great job taking care of me." Caring for him had been so hard on her, and John knew this and wanted his loving and faithful wife to be free of the struggle and from any remaining guilt she might be feeling.

John has now passed from this temporary life to experience eternal life. Despite having progressive dementia, through the working of the Spirit he spent his final days bringing peace to those he left behind. While John joins in the "boogie party," his family now spends time remembering him as a husband, father, and man of God. Though his final years were painful, certainly not what they expected, his wife testifies to the goodness of the Lord and the unexpected expressions of his grace in the most difficult of circumstances. "By God's grace, we were able to taste and see that the Lord is good!"

Death is not the end. Yes, it brings an end to dementia and the battle with Alzheimer's, and it also brings the promised end to our suffering. Because of Christ's suffering and resurrection we are promised that our suffering will come to an end, and God will bring us into his presence where all things are made new. Here we will know incomparable glory, enduring joy, true freedom from sin and decay, and restoration to the perfected image of God.[4]

We may doubt and forget, but God has not forgotten us or his promises.

> *O Lord,*
> *I live here as a fish in a vessel of water,*
> *   only enough to keep me alive,*
> *   but in heaven I shall swim in the ocean.*
> *Here I have a little air in me to keep me breathing,*
> *   but there I shall have sweet and fresh gales;*
> *Here I have a beam of sun to lighten my darkness,*
> *   a warm ray to keep me from freezing;*
> *   yonder I shall live in light and warmth forever.*
> *My natural desires are corrupt and misguided,*
> *   and it is thy mercy to destroy them;*
> *My spiritual longings are of thy planting,*
> *   and thou wilt water and increase them;*
> *Quicken my hunger and thirst after the realm above.*

Here I can have the world,
        there I shall have thee in Christ;
Here is a life of longing and prayer,
        there is assurance without suspicion,
        asking without refusal;
Here are gross comforts, more burden than benefit,
        there is joy without sorrow,
        comfort without suffering,
        love without inconstancy,
        rest without weariness.
Give me to know that heaven is all love,
        where the eye affects the heart,
        and the continual viewing of thy beauty
        keeps the soul in continual transports of delight.
Give me to know that heaven is all peace,
        where error, pride, rebellion, passion raise no head.
Give me to know that heaven is all joy,
        the end of believing, fasting, praying,
        mourning, humbling, watching, fearing, repining;
And lead me to it soon.[5]

AFTERWORD

ALZHEIMER'S IS ONE OF THE MOST FEARED DISEASES, and because it seems to attack the very core of our being, it can lead us to question how we think and live.

Alzheimer's forces us to reconsider the ways that we think about our relationship with God, our spiritual life, and how we minister to one another. It pushes us toward aspects of God's character that we may forget or neglect. In Alzheimer's care we are forced to lean more heavily on God's sovereignty, the ever-present working of his Spirit, and his incomprehensible grace in reaching the person who is in progressive decline. We are reminded that God reaches for us before we remember to reach for him. When we groan, the Lord hears, understands, and groans with us.

Alzheimer's also pushes our ministry to be less dependent upon words, to focus on grace in the present moment (even if it is later forgotten), to expand our view of remembering, and to trust that the person is held in the arms of a loving God who can penetrate even the depths of advanced dementia. We use words, but we also speak to the person through music, stories, and the kindness of our actions. We invite but do not expect them to remember later. We thank God for each moment of clarity as evidence of his sustaining grace! When it comes to faith, caregivers and family members are forced to trust more heavily the sovereignty and grace of God, who is the author and sustainer of our faith. Let us praise the Lord and not forget all of his benefits (Psalm 103).

• • •

Here are a few commonly asked questions:

How can I begin to minister to those with Alzheimer's or other dementias?

- Have a special message or a Sunday service dedicated to the theme of remembering and praying for those with Alzheimer's.
- Consider starting a support group or ministry for caregivers or for those struggling with Alzheimer's.
- Start a prayer meeting or hymn sing for people and families affected by Alzheimer's.
- Organize a group from your church for an event like the Walk to End Alzheimer's sponsored by the Alzheimer's Association *alz.org/walk.*
- *Above all,* seek to be present, show love, and remain with them on this journey.

Where can I learn more about Alzheimer's disease, its causes, and it treatment?

The Alzheimer's Disease Education and Referral Center (a branch of the National Institute on Aging) is an excellent source for current research and education materials, including some free publications. You can also find ongoing research studies and clinical trials through their website: *nia.nih.gov/alzheimers* or by calling 1-800-438-4380.

I highly recommend their publication entitled *Alzheimer's Disease: Unraveling the Mystery*, which is described as an "essential primer on Alzheimer's disease" and is updated annually: *nia.nih.gov/alzheimers/ publication/alzheimers-disease-unraveling-mystery.*

Where can I find help with caregiving? Care planning? Medical and legal planning for the future? Where can I find a support group?

The Alzheimer's Association has both national and local chapters that offer support, education, and a twenty-four-hour helpline for caregivers (1-800-272-3900). You can find local support groups, education programs, and other help through their national website: *alz.org/* or by calling the 24/7 helpline. Some local chapters may also be able to recommend a physician or psychologist to help with diagnosis and care planning.

Are there other books for caregivers that you would recommend?

I recommend books describing the "Best Friends Approach" developed by Virginia Bell and David Troxel. The most recent and updated is *A Dignified Life: The Best Friends Approach to Alzheimer's Care, A Guide for Family Caregivers* (Health Professions Press, 2012).

Joanne Brackey's *Creating Moments of Joy for the Person with Alzheimer's or Dementia: A Journal for Caregivers*, Fourth Edition (Lafayette, Ind.: Purdue University Press, 2008) is a helpful resource for living with and caring for a person with dementia, which focuses on living in the moment and creating opportunities to experience joy.

Robert Davis's *My Journey into Alzheimer's Disease: A True Story* (Carol Stream, Ill.: Tyndale House, 1989) is one pastor's account of his diagnosis and life with Alzheimer's disease and faith.

The 36-Hour Day: A Family Guide to Caring for People Who Have Alzheimer Disease, Related Dementias, and Memory Loss (New York: Grand Central Life and Style, 2012) by Nancy L. Mace and Peter C. Rabins is a classic, yet continually updated practical guide to understanding Alzheimer's disease and caregiving.

Where can I find more information on other types of dementia?

In addition to the Alzheimer's Association and National Institute on Aging websites (above), the University of California-San Francisco's Memory and Aging Center is a very helpful resource for further education on the various types of dementia: *memory.ucsf.edu/ education/diseases*.

ACKNOWLEDGMENTS

LIFE IS OFTEN BUSY, SOMETIMES CONFUSING, and marked by uncertainty. Occasionally we get a clear glimpse of what God is doing in our lives, and we are humbled to see how he weaves people and events together in mysterious ways that we could never have envisioned ahead of time. I first want to thank the Lord, and celebrate his goodness in bringing together all the people that helped make this book what it is today. You are the author of my faith and my life, I am so grateful that your ways and plans are much better than mine.

Thank you to the families who shared their experiences with me regarding their faith and the journey into and through Alzheimer's disease and other dementias. Your time, stories, and encouragement are evidence of God's grace in the midst of struggle and I am very grateful that you were willing to share with me so that I could share with others. Your devotion to your loved ones and the Lord is an excellent picture of living out one's faith.

I would like to thank those who were willing to offer helpful input at various stages of this project: Carole Spaeth, Deborah Cooper, Sarah Garwood, Todd Robertson, Robert Plummer, James Santos, Robert Cheong, Andrew Hassler, Chad Lewis, Stan Mast, Jason Read, Michael Morgan, Mike Cosper, and Daniel Montgomery.

I would also like to acknowledge the pastors from Sojourn Community Church whose teaching has continued to form my faith and theology over the past twelve years. There are many, but in particular I want to thank Kevin Jamison, Jeremy Linneman, Robert Cheong, Chad Lewis, Mike Cosper, and Daniel Montgomery. A special thank-you goes to Robert Plummer whose persistent interest in this project helped moved this book out of the idea stages and into something others could read. Sometimes you never know how far a little encouragement will go. I am also thankful for Ryan Pazdur and the rest of the Zondervan team for taking an interest in this project and helping it reach fruition.

I also want to acknowledge generous support from the Louisville Institute, whose grants program helped fund the research and writing of this book.

Finally, I would like to acknowledge the support and encouragement of my family, especially my loving wife, Kristin. I also want to thank the many friends who supported me with encouragement, prayer, and well-timed celebratory dinners. I trust that you know who you are.

God has blessed me beyond measure through you.

NOTES

Chapter 1: What Is the Second Forgetting?

1. They should talk about his commands as they go about their daily business, write them on their doorframes and tie them to their foreheads (Deuteronomy 6:4–9). There is much, as you will see, that the Bible offers us in terms of tools to remember. See chapter 9.

Chapter 2: Understanding Alzheimer's Disease

1. B. L. Plassman, K. M. Langa, G. G. Fisher, S. G. Heeringa, D. R. Weir, M. B. Ofstedal, et al. "Prevalence of Dementia in the United States: The Aging, Demographics, and Memory Study," *Neuroepidemiology* 29 (2007): 125–32.

2. The sequence of events described in these paragraphs is referred to as the *amyloid cascade hypothesis*. It is, as of this writing, the dominant theory of how Alzheimer's pathology begins and spreads throughout the brain, although there is some debate. The interested and motivated reader might consult Hardy and Selkoe, "The Amyloid Hypothesis of Alzheimer's Disease: Progress and Problems on the Road to Therapeutics," *Science* 297 (2002): 353–56. Also, C. R. Jack, et al., "Hypothetical Model of Dynamic Biomarkers of the Alzheimer's Pathological Cascade," *The Lancet Neurology* 9 (2010): 119–28.

3. R. A. Sperling, et al., "Toward Defining the Preclinical Stages of Alzheimer's Disease: Recommendations from the National Institute on Aging-Alzheimer's Association Workgroups on Diagnostic Guidelines for Alzheimer's Disease," *Alzheimer's and Dementia* 7 (2011): 280–92.

4. For Alzheimer's disease research centers and for clinical trials, go to the Alzheimer's Disease Education and Referral Center website: *nia.nih.gov/alzheimers* or call 1-800-438-4380. You can also find clinical trials through

the Alzheimer's Association's TrialMatch service: *alz.org/research/clinical_trials/find_clinical_trials_trialmatch.asp* or by calling 1-800-272-3900.

5. J. Birks, "Cholinesterase Inhibitors for Alzheimer's Disease," *Cochrane Database of Systematic Reviews* (2006); J. Rodda and A. Walker, "Ten Years of Cholinesterase Inhibitors," *International Journal of Geriatric Psychiatry* 24 (2009): 437–42.

6. See these links for more information on staging systems: *alz.org/alzheimers_disease_stages_of_alzheimers.asp; dementia.americangeriatrics.org/#signs*.

7. B. T. Mast, "Uncertainties in Dementia: What Do People with Dementia Experience? *Generations* 33 (2009): 30–36; B. T. Mast, "Methods for Assessing the Person with Alzheimer's Disease: Integrating Person-Centered and Diagnostic Approaches to Assessment," *Clinical Gerontologist* 35 (2012): 360–75.

Chapter 3: Remembering and Forgetting

1. For a basic primer on the memory systems see *scholarpedia.org/article/Multiple_memory_systems*.

2. This refers mainly to the early to middle stages. As individuals move into later stages with more severe dementia, recalling older memories becomes more difficult, and the details may become confused.

3. *hbo.com/alzheimers/memory-loss-tapes.html*.

4. Although these people didn't have Alzheimer's disease, they did have damage to the hippocampus (the primary brain structure affected in Alzheimer's) and had similar memory impairment.

5. J. S. Feinstein, M. C. Duff, and D. Tranel, "Sustained Experience of Emotion after Loss of Memory in Patients with Amnesia," *Proceedings of the National Academy of Sciences of the United States of America* 107 (2010): 7674–79.

6. L. R. Squire, "Memory Systems of the Brain: A Brief History and Current Perspective," *Neurobiology of Learning and Memory* 82 (2004): 171–77; H. L. Roediger, "Reconsidering Implicit Memory," in J. S. Bowers and C. Marsolek, eds., *Rethinking Implicit Memory* (London: Oxford University Press, 2003), 3–18.

Chapter 4: The Gospel for Those with Alzheimer's

1. MetLife Foundation, *MetLife Foundation Alzheimer's Survey: What America Thinks*, (New York: MetLife Foundation, 2006); B. T. Mast, "Methods for Assessing the Person with Alzheimer's Disease: Integrating Person-Centered and Diagnostic Approaches to Assessment," *Clinical Gerontologist* 35 (2012): 360–75.

2. John Swinton, *Dementia: Living in the Memories of God* (Grand Rapids, Mich.: Eerdmans, 2012).

3. Robert A. Peterson, "Suffering and the Biblical Story" in Christopher W. Morgan and Robert A. Peterson, eds., *Suffering and the Goodness of God* (Wheaton, Ill.: Crossway, 2008).

4. Ibid, 124.

5. Though the fall tells the story of how sin, suffering, and death entered the world, it does not address the more personal question of why specific individuals suffer. Though sin and suffering are linked in Genesis 3, the implication is not that your personal sin has caused your personal suffering. It is not fair or accurate to claim that any individual develops Alzheimer's because they sinned. I don't know anyone who claims or believes this. Alzheimer's is a reflection of this fallen world, rather than the result of some specific sin.

6. Peterson, "Suffering and the Biblical Story," 125.

7. Wayne Grudem, *Bible Doctrine: Essential Teachings of the Christian Faith.* (Grand Rapids, Mich.: Zondervan, 1999).

8. Graeme Goldsworthy, *According to Plan: The Unfolding Revelation of God in the Bible* (Downers Grove, Ill: IVP, 2002), 221.

9. See John Piper and Justin Taylor, *Suffering and the Sovereignty of God* (Wheaton, Ill.: Crossway, 2006) for a more general treatment of suffering.

10. D. L. Algase, C. Beck, A. Kolanowski, A. Whall, S. Berent, K. Richards, et al. "Need-Driven Dementia-Compromised Behavior: An Alternative View of Disruptive Behavior," *American Journal of Alzheimer's Disease and Other Dementias* 11 (1996): 10–19; C. R. Kovach, P. E. Noonan, A. M. Schlidt, and T. Wells, "A Model of Consequences of Need-Driven, Dementia-Compromised Behavior," *Journal of Nursing Scholarship* 37 (2005): 134–40.

11. B. T. Mast, *Whole Person Dementia Assessment.* (Baltimore: Health Professions, 2011).

12. J. I. Packer, *Knowing God* (Downers Grove, Ill.: InterVarsity, 1993), 41–42; *thegospelcoalition.org/blogs/justintaylor/2012/08/14/more-important-than-knowing-god/*.

Chapter 5: The Challenges of Giving Care

1. For a very helpful perspective on the busyness of life, see Kevin DeYoung, *Crazy Busy: A (Mercifully) Short Book about a (Really) Big Problem* (Wheaton, Ill.: Crossway, 2013).

2. Up to 60 percent of people with Alzheimer's disease wander at some point. Few who wander away from home can find their way home without help. See C. G. Lyketsos, O. Lopez, B. Jones, A. L. Fitzpatrick, J. Breitner, J., and S. DeKosky, "Prevalence of Neuropsychiatric Symptoms in Dementia and Mild Cognitive Impairment — Results from the Cardiovascular Health Study," *Journal of the American Medical Association* 288 (2002): 1475–83.

3. Michael Castleman, Dolores Gallagher-Thompson, and Matthew Naythons, *There's Still a Person in There* (New York: Perigee, 2000).

4. Ibid.

5. See S. H. Zarit and A. M. Reamy, "Assessment and Treatment of Family Caregivers," in P. A. Lichtenberg and B.T. Mast, eds., *APA Handbook of Clinical Geropsychology* (Washington, D.C: American Psychological Association, 2015).

6. Up to 90 percent at some point; *Generation Alzheimer's: the Defining Disease of the Baby Boomers* (Chicago, Ill: Alzheimer's Association), *alz.org/boomers/*.

7. I. S. Shin, M. Carter, D. Masterman, L. Fairbanks, and J. L. Cummings, "Neuropsychiatric Symptoms and Quality of Life in Alzheimer Disease," *American Journal of Geriatric Psychiatry* 13 (2005): 469–74.

8. C. K. Holley and B. T. Mast, "Predictors of Anticipatory Grief in Dementia Caregivers," *Clinical Gerontologist* 33 (2010): 223–36.

9. *The Sandwich Generation. Rising Financial Burdens for Middle Aged Americans* (Washington, D.C., Pew Research Center, January 2013). The full report can be found at *pewsocialtrends.org/files/2013/01/Sandwich_Generation_Report_FINAL_1–29.pdf*.

10. K. L. Fingerman, L. M. Pitzer, W. Chan, K. Birditt, M. M. Franks, and S. Zarit, "Who Gets What and Why? Help Middle-Aged Adults Provide to Parents and Grown Children," *The Journals of Gerontology Series B: Psychological Sciences and Social Sciences* 66B (2010): 87–98.

11. Randy Alcorn, "A Prayer of Weariness." Used by permission. *Eternal Perspective Ministries:* http://www.epm.org/resources/2010/Dec25/prayer-weariness/

Chapter 6: God's Grace for Caregivers

1. See the story of Robert McQuilkin as a notable exception: Robert McQuilkin, "Living by Vows," *Christianity Today* (February 2004), *christianitytoday.com/ct/2004/februaryweb-only/2–9–11.0.html*; and Robert McQuilkin, "Muriel's Blessing," *Christianity Today* (February 2004), *christianitytoday.com/ct/2004/februaryweb-only/2–9–12.0.html.*

2. Dietrich Bonhoeffer, *Life Together* (New York: Harper & Row, 1954), 99.

3. See Robert L. Plummer, *Forty Questions about Interpreting the Bible*, (Grand Rapids, Mich.: Kregel, 2010), 249–50.

4. With the exception, of course, of the day before the Sabbath.

5. Ann Voskamp, *One Thousand Gifts* (Grand Rapids, Mich.: Zondervan, 2011), 59.

6. Most likely, the person you care for doesn't want to be a burden to you either.

7. J. K. Kiecolt-Glaser, P. T. Marucha, A. M. Mercado, W. B. Malarkey, and R. Glaser, "Slowing of Wound Healing by Psychological Stress," *The Lancet* 346 (November 4, 1995): 1194–96.

8. Deborah Cooper, "Caring for the Caregiver," *The Southeast Outlook*, *southeastoutlook.org/living_strong/article_9fddbaae-0d5a-11e2-b963-001a4bcf6878.html* (posted October 3, 2012).

Chapter 7: Alzheimer's and the Church

1. B. L. Plassman, et al., "Prevalence of Dementia in the United States: The Aging, Demographics and Memory Study," *Neuroepidemiology* 29 (2007): 125–32; B. L. Plassman, et al, "Prevalence of Cognitive Impairment without Dementia in the United States," *Annals of Internal Medicine* 148 (2008): 427–34.
2. *Generation Alzheimer's: The Defining Disease of the Baby Boomers* (Chicago, Ill.: Alzheimer's Association, 2011), *alz.org/boomers/*
3. Hugh Halter and Matt Smay, *AND: The Gathered and Scattered Church*. (Grand Rapids, Mich.: Zondervan, 2011).
4. Mike Cosper, *Rhythms of Grace: How the Church's Worship Tells the Story of the Gospel* (Wheaton, Ill.: Crossway, 2013).
5. Stephen G. Post, *The Moral Challenge of Alzheimer's Disease* (Baltimore: Johns Hopkins University Press, 2000).
6. Wayne Grudem, *Bible Doctrine* (Grand Rapids, Mich.: Zondervan, 1999), 36.
7. Gregg R. Allison, *Sojourners and Strangers: The Doctrine of the Church* (Wheaton, Ill.: Crossway, 2012), 117–18.
8. See Susan H. McFadden and John T. McFadden, *Aging Together: Dementia, Friendship and Flourishing Communities* (Baltimore: Johns Hopkins University Press, 2011).

Chapter 8: Remembering Stories of Faith

1. R. N. Butler, "The Life Review: An Interpretation of Reminiscence in the Aged," *Psychiatry* 26 (1963): 65–76; B. K. Haight, D. L. Bachman, S. Hendrix, M. T. Wagner, A. Meeks, and J. Johnson, "Life Review: Treating the Dyadic Family Unit with Dementia," *Clinical Psychology and Psychotherapy* 10 (2003), 165–74; F. Scogin, D. Welsh, A. Hanson, J. Stump, and A. Coates, "Evidence-Based Psychotherapies for Depression in Older Adults," *Clinical Psychology-Science and Practice* 12 (2005): 222–37.
2. Craig G. Bartholomew and Michael W. Goheen, *The Drama of Scripture: Finding Our Place in the Biblical Story* (Grand Rapids, Mich.: Baker, 2004).
3. Steven R. Sabat, *The Experience of Alzheimer's Disease: Life through a Tangled Veil* (Hoboken, N.J.: Wiley-Blackwell, 2001).
4. B. K. Haight, F. Gibson, and Y. Michel, "The Northern Ireland Life Review/Life Storybook Project for People with Dementia," *Alzheimers and Dementia* 2 (2006): 56–58; B. K. Haight, D. L. Bachman, S. Hendrix,

M. T. Wagner, A. Meeks, and J. Johnson, "Life Review: Treating the Dyadic Family Unit with Dementia," *Clinical Psychology and Psychotherapy* 10 (2003): 165–74.

5. J. C. Stuckey, S. G. Post, S. Ollerton, S. J. FallCreek, and P. J. Whitehouse, "Alzheimer's Disease, Religion, and the Ethics of Respect for Spirituality," *Alzheimer's Care Quarterly* 3 (2002): 199–207.

6. These questions were adapted from several sources and I recommend these as additional resources: Corinne Trevitt and Elizabeth MacKinlay, " 'I Am Just an Ordinary Person ...': Spiritual Reminiscence in Older People with Memory Loss," *Journal of Religion, Spirituality and Aging* 18 (2006): 79–91; James M. Houston and Michael Parker, *A Vision for the Aging Church: Renewing Ministry for and by Seniors"* (Downers Grove, Ill." InterVarsity, 2011); Virginia Bell and David Troxel, *A Dignified Life: The Best Friends Approach to Alzheimer's Care, A Guide for Family Caregivers* (Deerfield Beach, Fla.: Health Communications, 2012); Benjamin Mast, *Whole Person Dementia Assessment* (Baltimore: Health Professions Press, 2011); Barbara K. Haight and Barrett S. Haight, *The Handbook of Structured Life Review* (Baltimore: Health Professions Press, 2007).

7. John Swinton, *Dementia: Living in the Memories of God* (Grand Rapids, Mich.: Eerdmans, 2012).

Chapter 9: Remembering the Lord

1. If you skipped chapter 3, it may be helpful to go back and read it before this chapter.

2. Donald Whitney, *Spiritual Disciplines for the Christian Life* (Colorado Springs: NavPress, 1997).

3. Mark Thompson, *A Clear and Present Word: The Clarity of Scripture* (Downers Grove, Ill.: InterVarsity, 2006).

4. Mike Cosper, *Rhythms of Grace: How the Church's Worship Tells the Story of the Gospel* (Wheaton, Ill.: Crossway, 2013).

5. Stan Mast, "And Heals All Your Diseases," *Catapult Magazine*, catapultmagazine.com/in-sickness/feature/and-heals-all-your-diseases.

6. A full treatment of Communion is beyond the scope of this book, but it should be noted that there are several Christian views on Communion that differ from the one presented here. The interested reader may consult the chapter on the Lord's Supper in Gregg R. Allison's *Sojourners and Strangers: The Doctrine of the Church* (Wheaton, Ill.: Crossway, 2012).

7. J. C. Stuckey, S. G. Post, S. Ollerton, S. J. FallCreek, and P. J. Whitehouse, "Alzheimer's Disease, Religion, and the Ethics of Respect for Spirituality," *Alzheimer's Care Quarterly* 3 (2002): 199–207.

8. Gregg R. Allison's *Sojourners and Strangers: The Doctrine of the Church* (Wheaton, Ill.: Crossway, 2012), 117.

Chapter 10: Prevention and Planning

1. The findings discussed, in fact, have been doubly reviewed, first in terms of peer review for publication in scientific journals, and second by a consensus panel convened by the U.S. National Institutes of Health.
2. NIH Consensus Panel, B. L. Plassman, et al, "Systematic Review: Factors Associated with Risk for and Possible Prevention of Cognitive Decline in Later Life," *Annals of Internal Medicine* 153 (2010): 182–93.
3. Metabolic syndrome refers to a clustering of several risk factors that increase risk for stroke and heart disease: a large waistline, high triglyceride level, low HDL level, high blood pressure and high fasting glucose; see this NIH site for more information: *nhlbi.nih.gov/health/health-topics/topics/ms/*.
4. J. S. Goldman, et al., "Genetic Counseling and Testing for Alzheimer's Disease: Joint Practice Guidelines of the American College of Medical Genetics and the National Society of Genetic Counselors," *Genetics in Medicine* 13 (2011): 597–605.
5. J. S. Roberts and S. M. Tersengo, "Estimating and Disclosing the Risk of Developing Alzheimer's Disease: Challenges, Controversies, and Future Directions," *Future Neurology* 5 (2010): 501–17.
6. R. S. Wilson, et al., "Loneliness and Risk of Alzheimer's Disease," *Archives of General Psychiatry* 63 (2007): 234–40.
7. See Hyer, et al. (in press). "Cognitive Training for Mildly Impaired Older Adults," in P. A. Lichtenberg and B. T. Mast, eds., *APA Handbook of Clinical Geropsychology* (Washington, D.C.: American Psychological Association).
8. *alz.org/alzheimers_disease_facts_and_figures.asp*.
9. The Alzheimer's Association has many helpful tips in their Caregiver Center (*alz.org/care/overview.asp*), including an "End of Life Decisions" document, which can be found at *alz.org/national/documents/brochure_endoflifedecisions.pdf*.
10. L. L. Carstensen, "The Influence of Sense of Time on Human Development," *Science* 312 (2006): 1913–15. And L. L. Carstensen, et al., "Taking Time Seriously: A Theory of Socioemotional Selectivity," *American Psychologist* 54 (1999): 165–81.
11. S. H. Zarit and A. M. Reamy, "Assessment and Treatment of Family Caregivers," in P. A. Lichtenberg and B. T. Mast, eds., *APA Handbook of Clinical Geropsychology* (Washington, D.C.: American Psychological Association, 2015).
12. N. T. Wright, *After You Believe: Why Christian Character Matters* (San Francisco: HarperOne, 2012), 20–21.
13. N. Archer, R. G. Brown, S. J. Reeves, H. Boothby, H. Nicholas, C. Foy, et al., "Premorbid Personality and Behavioral and Psychological Symptoms in Probable Alzheimer Disease," *American Journal of Geriatric Psychiatry* 15 (2007): 202–13.

14. See Donald S. Whitney's *Spiritual Disciplines for the Christian Life* (Colorado Springs: NavPress, 1997) for a helpful treatment of the spiritual disciplines.

15. John Piper, "Resolutions on Growing Old with God," *desiringgod.org /resource-library/taste-see-articles/resolutions-on-growing-old-with-god*, © 2013 Desiring God Foundation. Website: *desiringGod.org*.

Chapter 11: God Never Forgets

1. See also D. K. McKim, *God Never Forgets: Faith, Hope and Alzheimer's Disease* (Louisville: Westminster John Knox Press, 1997).

2. R. E. Van Voorst, "The Biblical Concept of Remembering and Ministry to People with Alzheimer's Disease," *Reformed Review* 54(2) (2001): 99–107.

3. Augustine, *Confessions*, Book 1, 1–2.

4. Christopher W. Morgan and Robert A. Peterson, eds., *Suffering and the Goodness of God* (Wheaton, Ill.: Crossway, 2008), 137–38.

5. Arthur G. Bennett, *Valley of Vision: A Collection of Puritan Prayers and Devotions* (Edinburgh: Banner of Truth, 2003), 370–71.

SUBJECT INDEX

SCRIPTURE INDEX